ANXIETY AND
NEUROTIC DISORDERS

APPROACHES TO
BEHAVIOR PATHOLOGY SERIES
Brendan Maher — Series Editor

ANXIETY AND NEUROTIC DISORDERS

BARCLAY MARTIN

RxTSA

John Wiley & Sons, Inc.

New York · London · Sydney · Toronto

Library of Congress Catalogue Card Number: 76-151033

ISBN   0-471-57350-7 (cloth)
ISBN   0-471-57353-1 (paper)

Printed in the United States of America

10   9   8   7   6   5   4   3   2   1

To My Parents and My Daughters,
Susan and Betsy

SERIES PREFACE

Abnormal psychology may be studied in many different ways. One traditional method of approach emphasizes the description of clinical syndromes with an extensive use of case histories to illustrate the central phenomena and the psychological processes believed to underlie them. Another common position is found in the adoption of a systematic theory (such as psychodynamic or behavioral) as a framework within which important problems of abnormal psychology may be delineated and interpreted.

Whether systematic or eclectic, descriptive or interpretive, the teaching of a course in abnormal psychology faces certain difficult problems. Just as in other areas of science, abnormal psychology has exhibited a rapid increase in knowledge and in the rate at which new knowledge is being acquired. It is becoming more and more difficult for the college teacher to keep abreast of contemporary developments over as wide a range of subjects as abnormal psychology encompasses. Even in the areas of his personal interest and special competence the instructor may be hard pressed to cover significant concepts and findings with real comprehensiveness.

Adding to this spate of new knowledge is the fact that, in the field of abnormal psychology, we are witnessing a resurgence of enthusiasm for empirical research of an experimental kind together with a growth of interest in deviant behavior on the part of other scientists, notably the geneticists, neurobiologists, biochemists on the one hand and epidemiologists, anthropologists and social scientists on the other. It is less and less possible to claim mastery of a topic area in abnormal psychology when approaching it purely from the standpoint of a single psychological theory. An adequate understanding of any central topic now depends on familiarity with literature coming from many quarters of the scientific community.

Knowledge multiplies but time does not. Working within the limits of forty to fifty lecture hours available for the usual course in general abnormal psychology, it has become necessary for the student to turn more and more often to specialized outside reading to acquire the depth that cannot be given by any one textbook or by any one instructor. Although much can be gained by reading a range of selected reprints, these are often written originally for audiences other than the undergraduates and for purposes too narrowly technical to be entirely suited to instruction.

The present volume is one of a series developed to meet the need for depth of coverage in the central topic areas of abnormal psychology. The series is prepared with certain criteria in mind. Each volume has been planned to be scientifically authoritative, to be written with the clarity and directness necessary for the introductory student, but with a sophistication and timeliness of treatment that should render it of value to the advanced student and the fellow-specialist. Selection of the topics to be included in the series has been guided by a decision to concentrate on problem areas that are systematically and empirically important: in each case there are significant theoretical problems to be examined and a body of research literature to cast light on the several solutions that are adduced. Although it is anticipated that the student may read one or more of these volumes in addition to a standard text, the total series will cover the major part of a typical course in abnormal psychology and could well be used in place of a single text.

We are in a period of exciting growth and change in abnormal psychology. Concepts and hypotheses that have dominated the field for over half a century are giving place to new and provocative viewpoints. Much of this has been accomplished in one short decade: it is clear that the character of the field will be changed even more radically in the decades to come. It is the hope of the editor and the contributors to this series that they will play a useful part in preparing the coming generation of psychopathologists for the challenge of the years that lie ahead.

BRENDAN MAHER

PREFACE

Almost a hundred years have passed since Sigmund Freud started the movement that was to popularize terms such as anxiety and neurosis. A century of clinical study and systematic research has markedly increased our understanding of these disorders, and writing this book has stimulated me to organize my own thinking about the current status of knowledge in this area. One thing has become clear as a result of this effort: much remains to be learned. It is easy to give lip service to the abstraction that neurotic disorders result from an interplay of biological (including genetic) factors, past environmental influences, and present circumstances. A major aim of this book is to review the evidence on the contribution of these factors. There is a great and continuing need, however, for direct studies of the developmental processes themselves as they are involved in the production of neurotic disorders.

There is a strong current of antiscientism these days. I hear students complaining that psychology is "too scientific," and many professional psychologists have identified themselves as humanistic psychologists as opposed to scientific or research-oriented psychologists. The core of the disenchantment with psychological science seems to center around the assertion that scientifically oriented psychologists perceive people as objects to be studied and analyzed, and not as persons to be understood and appreciated in a holistic and nonanalytic sense. We cannot discount the possibility that preoccupation with science and technology in our society may have contributed more to a rapid development of such things as nuclear bombs and automobiles than to our capacity to prevent self-destruction and environmental pollution from these devices.

Students beginning the study of behavior pathology should be made aware, however, that there is no inherent incompatibility between the acquisition of scientific knowledge about human behavior and the espousal of humanistic values. Certainly the development of the Salk vaccine for poliomyelitis—the result of much tedious analytical research—has resulted in the implementation of a great humanistic value: the prevention of this crippling disease. It is my hope that a greater understanding of human psychological functioning (in particular, an understanding of neurotic disorders) will enable us to free ourselves from this kind of suffering—a freedom that we have not yet fully achieved.

The preparation of this book and some of the research cited herein were supported in part by the United States Department of Health, Education and Welfare, National Institute of Mental Health research grant MH 12474, and in part by the University of Wisconsin Graduate School Research Committee. Part of the manuscript was written while I was associated with the Oregon Research Institute, Eugene, Oregon, and I thank Paul Hoffman, Director of O.R.I., for the use of those facilities. I thank Mrs. Judy Boylan and Mrs. Shirley Harless for their patience and care in typing the manuscript; Mrs. Arlen Sue Fox of Wiley for her most helpful editorial assistance; and my wife, Liz, for reading and commenting on the early drafts of the manuscript.

Barclay Martin

CONTENTS

ANXIETY AND
NEUROTIC DISORDERS

CHAPTER ONE

INTRODUCTION

AN ILLUSTRATION

Twenty-five-year-old Harvey A. was a man with superior intelligence (verbal I.Q. over 130 as estimated from a short form of the Wechsler Adult Intelligence Scale) when he sought help at a psychological clinic. He had performed poorly in high school and had to repeat his junior year. After graduation, he held a succession of temporary jobs for a year or two, and then enrolled in, and successfully completed, two years of a junior college. He was subsequently admitted to a state university, where he experienced great difficulty with his academic work. He spent long hours in inefficient studying, read very slowly, and was particularly distressed by a severe difficulty in spelling. A course in remedial spelling did no good. Harvey A. dropped out of school after a year, and has since held a number of unskilled jobs.

He has had as many difficulties in his social relations as in the academic and vocational areas. His father died when he was 14. Shortly thereafter his mother began to have a series of affairs that eventuated in a brief marriage to a man who was apparently an alcoholic. This stepfather was belligerent and assaultive when drunk, and Harvey recalled several incidents in which his mother called on him to protect her from the stepfather's rages. In one instance a physical fight ensued in which Harvey knocked the older man down. Following his mother's divorce from this man and a period of further instability in the family situation he moved in

1

with his recently married older sister. For a short while he experienced a more relaxing home situation, obtaining "more mothering from my sister than I ever got from my mother."

More currently Harvey reports generalized feelings of tension and apprehension. He is especially sensitive to being jeered or laughed at by working men such as construction workers. He has a mustache, and this results in his being the occasional target of taunts of this kind directed by working men toward university students. He and his roommate were also pushed around a bit by four marines one night, and Harvey has since been very fearful of walking the streets after dark.

His relationship with his roommate has been a source of some distress. Harvey fears that his roommate could "destroy" him, if he chose to do so, by a sustained verbal assault. He has dated several girl friends, and has a continuing involvement with one including sexual relations. He nevertheless is apprehensive about his relationship with this girl, and worries that she may reject him.

On a checklist of fears he reported strong fear of being alone, speaking in public, failure, one person bullying another, being criticized, being rejected by others, being disapproved by others, making mistakes, and looking foolish.

In summary, Harvey A. presented a picture of chronic inability to master academic and vocational goals, chronic difficulty in achieving satisfying interpersonal relationships, and continuing fearfulness in many situations that seem to have in common a potential for criticism and ridicule. In addition, he reports feelings of loneliness, discouragement, and depression—hardly surprising in view of the above.

QUESTIONS TO BE ANSWERED

If we assume that Harvey does have high intelligence, basically good physical health, and motivation to achieve satisfying vocational and interpersonal goals, how can we explain his obvious inability to do so? A basic aim of this book is to bring together the current knowledge relevant to this question and attempt a scientific answer. The answer will not be complete. The question has many parts, and some of these parts must await further research before they can be answered in detail. Nevertheless, the body of clinical and research literature has been increasing steadily over the years, and it is becoming more and more possible to develop, at least in broad outline, a convincing portrayal of the nature and causation of neurotic disorders.

One conclusion might as well be stated at the outset. Neurosis is a multidetermined phenomenon. In any given case, such as that of Harvey A., the nature and severity of neurotic disorder is likely to be the result of three factors: hereditary dispositions, history of past experiences that would affect learned reactions or biological systems, and current situational factors. The weight given to any one of these factors will vary from individual to individual; it may be that hereditary tendencies are of little significance and past learning experiences are most important in one case, whereas in another case current situational factors, as in certain war neuroses, may be most influential. If this conclusion is warranted, it follows that there will be no simple answers to questions such as, "Is neurosis inherited?" or "Is neurosis the result of family experiences in the first five years of life?"

WHAT IS A NEUROTIC DISORDER?

In a sense the entire book is devoted to answering this question. The use of one term, neurosis, implies that we are dealing with a single entity. In fact, it is preferable to think of a broad spectrum of disorders, caused by a variety of biosocial factors, that are grouped under the heading of neurotic disorders. These disorders blend without sharp boundaries into "normality" on one hand and various other types of psychopathology, such as psychosomatic disorders, character disorders, and psychotic disorders on the other hand. The phenomenon of neurotic disorder simply does not lend itself to highly specific definition as, for example, do the disorders of a broken leg or a peptic ulcer. In broad outline it may be conceived as a handicap in psychological functioning that has its locus in emotional and interpersonal aspects of behavior.

Handicap is used in its everyday meaning; that is, a person is unable to do certain things that he would otherwise be able to do. The person frequently, but not always, reports subjective distress as an accompaniment to his difficulties. The handicap would not ordinarily be considered neurotic if it were a direct result of physical disorder, low intelligence, or coercive external circumstances such as being in prison. The important point here is that the person is *unable* to do or avoid certain things, not that he simply does not do them or avoids them. Dropping out of college is not in itself a neurotic response, but when, as in the case of Harvey A., the person apparently wants to continue, has the necessary intelligence, physical health, and so on, but is nevertheless unable to continue then it may reflect a neurotic disorder.

Statistical deviation approaches to the definition of neurotic disorder are unsatisfactory, and will be dismissed without much elaboration. Suffice it to say that a person's behaving in an unusual way does not make him neurotic. Such a simple-minded approach would label all concert pianists, ball players with batting averages over .300, and Nobel Prize winners as neurotic!

Nor will we consider society's evaluation of behavior as good or bad as being very important in deciding whether the behavior is defined as neurotic. Some individuals with severe neurotic handicaps behave in exemplary fashion according to society's code of ethics, and other individuals who flagrantly violate society's standards, certain professional criminals, for example, should not be considered as neurotic at all by our "handicap" definition.

The looseness of our definition of neurotic disorder, then, in part reflects the wide variation in the phenomenon itself and, at its boundaries, the difficulty in sharply discriminating it from "normality" or other disorders. This looseness should not be taken as in any way questioning the reality of these disorders. They are real and pervasive. In an epidemiological study Srole et al. (1962) interviewed and administered a questionnaire to a random sample of 1660 individuals living in Manhattan's East Side. Symptoms indicative of mental disorder were measured and the percentage of individuals falling in six categories representing degree of impairment were as follows: Well, 18.5%; Mild, 36.3%; Moderate, 21.8%; Marked, 13.2%; Severe, 7.5%, and Incapacitated, 2.7%. Combining the last three categories, we find 23.4% of the sample was considered to have at least a marked degree of psychological handicap. The authors concluded that the disorders of about two-thirds of these individuals would be considered neurotic in nature—about 15.7% of the total sample. Similar results have been obtained in other epidemiological studies (Pasamanick, 1961; Philips, 1966). Even if the prevalence of neurotic disorder in the United States were only half the value indicated by this sample, which would almost certainly be an underestimate, there would be approximately 15 million people experiencing this handicap. The loss in manpower to society is staggering. The cost in human suffering to the person and those close to him cannot be measured.

SCIENTIFIC STUDY OF NEUROTIC DISORDER

Most of us would agree that "understanding human nature" is a good thing. However, when scientists actually begin to pursue this goal and make some progress, it can become a frightening prospect. It can be disturbing to think that human behavior is as lawfully determined as other scientific subject matter, such as the behavior of molecules or amoeba; and may someday be subject to a high degree of prediction and control. Nevertheless, we make that assumption in studying neurotic disorders.

A pitfall that many people, including some psychologists and others who should know better, fall into is "explaining" a phenomenon by giving it a name. One can achieve a certain sense of "explanation" by answering the question "Why do rocks fall to the ground?" by saying "because of gravity." Although for some people gravity might be a shorthand expression for a whole system of physical laws relating strength of gravitational attraction, mass, distance, etc., for most of us it is little more than a shorthand expression for the fact that rocks fall to the ground, and therefore has added nothing new to our understanding of the phenomenon.

In psychology a version of the "explaining by naming" game that is particularly troublesome is one in which we "explain" some aspect of human behavior by postulating some inner and unobservable mental state. "He went to the drinking fountain because he was *thirsty*." "He kicked the chair because he was *mad*." "Harvey A. dropped out of school because he was *anxious*." The italicized word in each statement refers to a hypothetical mental state that is supposed to explain the observed behavior, but in most cases the only evidence for the postulated mental event is the overt behavior, and the resulting statements are tautological. He kicked the chair because he was mad, and we know he was mad because he kicked the chair.

Although some psychologists, for this and related reasons, avoid postulating any hypothetical internal states in accounting for human behavior, most psychologists are willing to make some inferences about intervening events in their theorizing. A theory of this kind can be useful if it suggests new relationships and lines of research that the investigator might not otherwise have considered. The results of such research can then lead to the abandonment of the theory or its modification. To say that a person drinks because he is thirsty adds nothing to our understanding unless we develop a theory about the internal mechanisms of thirst that lead to illuminating experiments of this kind.

In the realms of human emotion, motivation, personality, and behavior disorder there is always a great danger of falling into the "explaining by naming" trap. Our every day language habits make it almost inevitable that we phrase things in this way. The critical question is whether one can, when challenged, show how the "explanation" really does suggest relationships that can be tested. I am almost certain to express myself in this way in the chapters ahead; you may wish to question in my use of terms such as anxiety, reinforcement, thoughts, and depression whether I am explaining something by giving it a name.

The overall goal of this book, then, is to appraise current knowledge with respect to the nature and development of neurotic disorder. Where knowledge is incomplete I shall attempt to identify problems, or state puzzles, that require answers, and in some cases present formulations that hopefully will suggest fruitful lines of empirical research.

REFERENCES

Pasamanick, B. A survey of mental disease in an urban population. IV: An approach to total prevalence rates. *Arch. gen. Psychiat.,* 1961, **5,** 151–155.

Philips, D. L. The "true prevalence" of mental illness in a New England state. *Community mental health Journal,* 1966, **2,** 35–40.

Srole, L., Langner, T. S., Michael, S. T., Opler, M. K., & Rennie, T. A. C. *Mental health in the metropolis. Midtown Manhattan study.* Vol. I. New York: McGraw-Hill, 1962.

CHAPTER TWO

SYMPTOMS OF NEUROTIC DISORDER

In this chapter common symptom patterns of neurotic disorder will be summarized according to the following traditional categories: anxiety reaction, phobic reaction, obsessive-compulsive reaction, hysterical reaction, and depressive reaction. This is a rather arbitrary grouping, and few patients fit neatly into any of the categories; many show combinations of symptoms, or symptoms unique to their case. Labeling a person with one of these terms is not important, and has only minimal implications for understanding or treating the disorder. The traditional categories, however, still provide a basis for systematic description of common neurotic symptomatology.

ANXIETY REACTION

Many physiological reactions are associated with anxiety, such as rapid heart rate, rapid or irregular breathing, and dizziness. These will be elaborated in the next chapter. In addition, a person is likely to report feelings of apprehension, vague expectations of impending disaster, or more specific fears of losing control, going to pieces, going insane, or dying. He is likely to experience insomnia, restlessness, recurring nightmares or anxiety dreams, difficulty in concentration, forgetfulness, physical fatigue, and general inefficiency in work or study. He is frequently irritable and somewhat depressed about his condition. The patient can see no rational explanation for the reaction, no real dangers that could account for such an extreme fear.

Against a background of chronic anxiety, individuals may experience periods of acute anxiety that last from a few minutes to an hour or more, and vary in frequency from several times a day to once every six months or longer. Harvey A. seems to have experienced mild to moderate anxiety in a chronic fashion.

A classic self-report description of an acute anxiety attack and the person's subsequent development of a phobic fear of going any distance from his home is provided by Leonard (1927).

> . . . . I take off my hat; I mop my head; I fan my face. Sinking . . . Isolation . . . diffused premonitions of horror. 'Charlie' . . . no answer. The minutes pass. 'Charlie, Charlie' . . . louder . . . and no answer. I am alone, alone, in the universe. Oh, to be home . . . home. 'Charlie.' Then on the tracks from behind Eagle Heights and the woods across the lake comes a freight-train, blowing its whistle. Down the same track. Less than an hour after the passenger-train. Instantaneously diffused premonitions become acute panic. The cabin of that locomotive *feels* right over my head, as if about to engulf me. I am obsessed with a *feeling* as of a big circle, hogshead, cistern-hold, or what not, in air just in front of me. The train *feels* as if it were about to rush over me. In reality it chugs on. I race back and forth on the embankment. I say to myself (and aloud): 'It is half a mile across the lake—it can't touch you, it can't; it can't run you down—half a mile across the lake.'. . . . . I am running round and round in a circle shrieking, when Charlie emerges from the woods.

With Charlie's help he manages to return home, where he reports the following:

> Charlie goes inside with me. My parents are there. I lie on the davenport. I shake with terror. I say in a low voice: 'Father and mother, this looks like the end. I guess I am dying.' Charlie tiptoes about, lowering the shades. The spell passes. But my father does not go down town to take part in the dedication of the Parish House . . being 'needed at home.' I sleep long that night. In the morning, though feeling strangely weak in body, I start out on a little walk down the street. Within a hundred feet of the house I am compelled to rush back, in horror of being so far away . . . a hundred feet away . . . from home and security. I have never walked or ridden, alone or with others, as a normal man since that day.
>
> For the emotion in the distance-phobia, as for the emotion in all others, there have been clearly defined degrees of intensity. Let me assume that I am walking down University Drive by the Lake. I am a normal man for the first quarter of a mile; for the next hundred yards I am in a mild state of dread,

controllable and controlled; for the next twenty yards in an acute state of dread, yet controlled; for the next ten, in an anguish of terror that hasn't reached the crisis of explosion; and in a half-dozen steps more I am in as fierce a panic of isolation from help and home and in immediate death as a man overboard in mid-Atlantic or on a window-ledge far up in a skyscraper with flames lapping his shoulders.

. . . the seizure leaves me always far more exposed to phobic seizures for weeks or months; increases my fear of the Fear; and, as in the distance-phobia, robs me of a goodly part of what little freedom of movement on street and hillside I have (selections from pp. 304–308).

PHOBIC REACTION

The major distinction to be made between the anxiety reaction and the phobic reaction is that in the former the anxiety response is pervasive. In the phobic reaction the anxiety is only elicited by a restricted class of stimuli, the phobic object or situation. Depending upon the ubiquity of the phobic stimuli the person may or may not experience frequent anxiety. In any case the anxiety will almost certainly be experienced less often than in an anxiety reaction. The distinction, nevertheless, is a relative one. Patients diagnosed with anxiety reaction almost always experience more severe anxiety in some situations than others, and rarely are they chronically anxious in all situations.

As is the case for most neurotic symptomatology milder forms of phobic fear occur in the normal range of experience. Some degree of irrational fear of heights, spiders, or small enclosures, for example, are common. It used to be fashionable to give a separate name to each fear eliciting stimulus: acrophobia, fear of high places; agoraphobia, fear of open places; claustrophobia, fear of closed places. The medical context in which these diagnostic labels were used suggested that different "diseases" were involved. Psychological analysis, however, indicates that the important feature is the attachment of fear to certain stimuli; since almost any stimulus can come to serve as a phobic stimulus, there is limited value in making up a new name for each.

It may turn out that certain classes of phobia have functional properties that warrant their separate consideration. Several studies (e.g., Lader, 1967) have suggested that phobias tend to fall into two relatively distinct categories: those having social implications and usually less tied to highly specific situations; and those involving highly specific and essentially non-social situations. Examples of the former are fears of leaving home, walking along streets, crowds, and speaking before audiences; they usually involve fear about leaving some source of interpersonal support or encountering some unpleasant interpersonal situation. Nonsocial phobic stimuli are animals (dogs, spiders, birds, etc.), hospitals, blood, accidents, heights, fire, weapons, and thunderstorms.

OBSESSIVE-COMPULSIVE REACTION

Obsessions are thoughts that intrude repeatedly into awareness. They are usually experienced as irrational, "unwanted," and difficult to control or stop. Compulsions are actions that one feels compelled to perform, and are likewise experienced as irrational and difficult to control. As in anxiety and phobic reactions, mild forms of obsessive-compulsive experience are not uncommon in normal individuals. A song we cannot get out of our mind, or a compulsion to return home to make sure that the door is locked or the stove turned off, when there is no rational basis to expect otherwise, are examples from everyday life. The distinction between obsession and compulsion is not particularly important. An obsessive thought, such as the idea that the stove was left on, frequently occurs as part of the compulsive act.

When obsessions and compulsions reach a neurotic degree of severity, they frequently reflect conflicting tendencies within the person. Aggressive or sexual thoughts may, for example, alternate with thoughts or actions that seem designed to counteract or inhibit them. Obsessive thoughts that would conflict with a person's usual standards of behavior might be: the idea of stabbing, choking, poisoning, shooting or otherwise injuring one's child, parent, spouse, sibling or self; the idea of shouting obscene words at home, work, or church; the wish that someone were dead, or the image of the person dying a horrible death; the thought or image of a forbidden sexual adventure, perhaps involving "perverted" sex acts; the thought of committing suicide by jumping out a window, or into the path of a truck; the thought of catching some disease if one touches doorknobs, bannisters, toilets, or other objects in public places. Counteracting thoughts or actions can be almost any kind of thinking ritual that distracts one from the disturbing thought, such as counting to oneself, counting telephone poles from a moving car, reciting certain words or phrases to oneself, or more elaborate verbal rituals that may have a scientific, philosophical or religious basis; cleanliness rituals; excessive politeness or courteousness; excessive orderliness and neatness in housekeeping or at the office; excessive attempts to schedule activities on a precise timetable.

Cameron (1963) provides an illustration of the emergence of a disturbing obsessive thought and the subsequent development of counteractive measures in a 42-year-old mother of three children.

She was serving the family dinner one evening when she dropped a dish on the table and smashed it. The accident appalled her. While clearing up the fragments she was seized with an unreasonable fear that bits of glass might get into her husband's food and kill him. She would not allow the meal to proceed until she had removed everything and reset the table with fresh linen and clean dishes. After this her fears, instead of subsiding, reached out to include intense anxiety over the possibility that she herself and her children might be killed by bits of glass (p. 384).

Subsequently during psychotherapy it was learned that some time before breaking the glass dish she had discovered that her husband was having an affair. She had felt humiliated and angered but had said nothing about it. When the dish had smashed she had momentarily been aware of the wish that he would eat glass and die.

In this case the obsessive thought seems to have occurred in clear awareness only once and thereafter the counteractive compulsions predominated. As time went by they became more and more extensive. She had to examine minutely each piece of glassware, and if it had the slightest chip in it she threw it away. She was compelled to carry it to the trash can herself to ensure that it was removed from the house, and she would then conduct an exhaustive search for the missing chip. She vaguely remembered reading that copper and aluminum pots were not safe for certain kinds of cooking and avoided using them. It occurred to her that her ring had copper in it so she took it off whenever she cooked or washed dishes. She began to worry about other kinds of danger such as the spread of virus disease from toilet to kitchen, contamination from pesticides and fertilizers used on the lawn. Further countermeasures included isolating all potential poisons in the garage, even cleaning fluids and scouring powders.

This case illustrates the close relationship between phobic fears and obsessive-compulsive symptoms. The woman's fear of chipped glass, virus infection, and pesticide contamination could appropriately be called phobias. The presence of the elaborate rituals designed to reduce these phobic fears associated with the obsessive wish to kill her husband leads to the obsessive-compulsive label.

Two other characteristics common in obsessive-compulsive disorder are indecisiveness and highly controlled emotions. The indecision is a consequence of strong conflicting tendencies. The woman described above might begin to set the table but then start to worry that the dishes had been improperly washed. She might vacillate back and forth for several minutes before finally giving in to the compulsion and rewashing the dishes. Some individuals become almost completely incapacitated by endless compulsive rituals and the immobilization associated with obsessive indecision and doubting.

Sometimes the excessive inhibition of emotional expression is reflected in the obsessive ideas and compulsive acts being experienced in a cold, detached and unemotional fashion. Lack of emotional spontaneity is also associated with excessive patterns of orderly, timetable living, and in the formal manner of interpersonal relations.

Stable obsessive-compulsive characteristics that develop over a long period of time can become more like personality traits than acute symptoms. Thus some individuals maintain with a great deal of rigidity well-ordered routines at work, home, and leisure. Such a person is likely to be concerned about neatness, symmetrical arrangement of material at his desk, pictures that do not hang straight, and punctuality.

In some cases the compulsive act, instead of being a countermeasure against socially unacceptable thoughts or actions, is itself a socially unacceptable act such as promiscuous or deviant sexual behavior, excessive eating, use of alcohol or other drugs, stealing (kleptomania), and fire setting (pyromania). Compulsions of this kind are sometimes discussed under headings other than neurosis; they may be called character disorders, addictions, or sexual deviations. Many factors can contribute to the development of behavior that is contrary to current social standards. When these behaviors have the quality of an irrational compulsion that is contrary to an individual's verbalized desires, I will consider them to be neurotic in nature.

HYSTERIA

The term hysteria has a long history dating back to ancient Greece where the disorder was thought to be caused by a wandering uterus. In the past the label has been more frequently applied to women than men; the specific symptoms, however, are by no means limited to women. A typical pattern involves many bodily symptoms that come and go in irregular fashion and considerable incapacitation in carrying out responsibilities at work or at home. It has become customary to subdivide the symptoms of hysteria into two classes, referred to as conversion and dissociative reactions.

Conversion Reaction

This term refers to bodily symptoms that primarily involve the skeletal musculature and sensory functions such as the following: partial or complete paralyses of the arms, legs, or other body parts; anesthesias or analgesias (parts of the body lose the sense of touch or pain, respectively); disturbances in vision and hearing, including partial or complete blindness or deafness; disturbances in speech, including complete mutism and aphonia (one can speak only in a whisper); "lump in the throat"; persistent coughing, belching, or sneezing; or muscular twitches called tics; the simulation of false symptoms of pregnancy. The term derives from the psychoanalytic theory that psychic energy is "converted" into a bodily symptom. I use the term only as a descriptive label for a class of symptoms with no theoretical assumptions implied.

The term *psychosomatic disorder* is reserved for bodily symptoms involving the autonomic nervous system, such as stomach ulcers, high blood pressure, diarrhea, and skin disturbances. Some symptoms such as headache, dysmenorrhea, vomiting, loss of appetite, and sexual disturbances such as impotence, premature ejaculation, or frigidity are sometimes called conversion and sometimes called psychosomatic symptoms. These distinctions in labeling may turn out to be of little significance. The thing to be emphasized in both conversion and psychosomatic symptoms is that psychological factors have played an important role in their development.

Dissociative Reaction

This term refers to departures from normal states of consciousness, and derives from the idea of one part of the "mind" or consciousness splitting off or becoming dissociated from another part. One type of dissociative reaction, *amnesia,* involves the loss of memory for past experiences. Typically during an amnesic episode a person cannot remember his name, where he lives, or anything about his life circumstances. He does not recognize friends or relatives. The amnesic period may last for an hour or two, or may last for years. When the person "returns" to his normal state of consciousness he does not usually remember much, if anything, about the episode. The *fugue (flight) reaction* is similar to amnesia except that there is a real flight from the present situation. The person frequently goes to some other part of the country, and may start an entirely new life, getting a job, marrying, and having children, in complete forgetfulness of an earlier life involving another job and family. *Multiple-personality* symptoms are rare, but involve an extension of the amnesic or fugue picture to one in which separate and different personalities develop within the same person. The person may then alternate among the two or more personalities with varying degrees of awareness of what transpires in the others.

Somnambulism

Sleepwalking is also considered a kind of dissociative reaction. After going to sleep the person arises during the night and engages in some kind of activity, usually rather aimless. He may or may not return to bed on his own. If he awakens naturally or in response to other people, he will not remember the somnambulistic period. Fits or convulsions that closely simulate epileptic seizures are also a variant of dissociative reaction.

Historical Development

It was through the study of conversion and dissociative reactions that the role of psychological factors in neurotic disorders received its primary impetus. In the late 19th century the French psychiatrist Charcot and his colleagues demonstrated how hysterical symptoms of this kind could frequently be modified, at least temporarily, by hypnotic suggestion, and also how hysterical symptoms could be induced in normal individuals by posthypnotic suggestion. He also pointed out that many hysterical symptoms did not make neurological sense. "Glove" anesthesias, for example, involved a loss of feeling in the hand covering the same area as a glove; there is no possible combination of neurological injuries that would result in this kind of anesthesia. Normal neurological reflexes in otherwise paralyzed limbs, or epileptic-like seizures in which patients uncannily fell in ways so as to not hurt themselves were further indications that the symptom was not caused by neurological disease. Charcot also described a common feature associated with hysterical symptoms: a lack of normal concern about the symptom and its possible implications, an attitude sometimes referred to as *la belle indifference*. Despite these various intimations of psychological causation Charcot was inclined to believe that some constitutional weakness of the central nervous system was a prerequisite for hysterical disorder.

Freud studied for a year with Charcot and was considerably influenced by him. Shortly thereafter Freud collaborated with Breuer (1953) in the study of the case of Fraulein Anna O. Anna O. had a number of hysterical symptoms, including paralysis of the neck muscles, right leg, and arm, as well as impairments in sight and hearing and frequent altered states of consciousness. Under hyponosis it was discovered that she had nursed her dying father and was in constant attendance at his bedside. One night she had dozed off and dreamed that a snake was attacking her father. She attempted to knock it away with her right hand but this hand had fallen asleep and would not move. The next day she reached into some bushes for a quoit, a branch reminded her of a snake, and her right arm became paralyzed. Breuer discovered that having her reexperience incidents of this sort with complete emotional expression often resulted in remission of the symptom. The case was considerably more complicated than this, but the excerpt provides the flavor of the kind of clinical evidence that set Freud on the road to theories of psychological causation of neuroses that were to eventuate in the movement known as psychoanalysis.

An Illustrative Case of Conversion Reaction

In both conversion and dissociative reactions it is usually apparent (not necessarily to the patient) that some acutely disturbing life situation is instrumental in precipitating the symptoms, as illustrated in the following case described by Carter (1937). Kate Fox, 13½ years of age, was admitted to the hospital with a partial paralysis of the left leg, extreme nervousness, and marked loss of appetite. When questioned on admission about the cause of these difficulties, she had no explanation. Her mother attributed the recent worsening of the symptoms to fright produced when a dog attacked Kate's sister. The symptoms, however, had been intermittently present for some time before the dog incident.

In a later interview, after some initial denial that there were any problems at home, she finally broke down and with much sobbing and trembling told the following story. Three years before her mother began an affair with a roomer in the house and eventually ran away with him. Within a few days the father and Kate and her three sisters found her and persuaded her to return home. A violent and abusive scene followed their arrival home in which Kate came to understand more clearly what her mother had done, and heard her mother accuse her father of running around with another woman. Nightly quarrels of this kind continued for several weeks and were very upsetting to Kate and her sisters. The parents at one point decided on a divorce, but one of the older sisters threatened suicide when she heard of this, and the parents changed their minds. At this time the former roomer returned and took residence across the street. The father threatened to shoot him if he came on the premises. A short time later a friend of the former roomer threatened to shoot her father and a fight ensued. Following this disturbance the parents agreed not to separate, for the sake of the children, and on the surface at least things seemed to go more smoothly in the home.

Kate reported that after these stressful episodes she could not bear to think of them, and became more and more withdrawn and uncommunicative at home. She found school a relief but within about a year began to develop a fear of social relationships at school. She would concentrate on her studies, grow fearful as recess time approached, and would frequently remain at her desk and study when the other children went out to play. Her initial paralysis came on just before a recess period.

The therapist, by urging her to retell, over and over again, the story of the painful episodes, was able to effect a complete removal of her symptoms within several weeks. At each successive retelling the emotional distress associated with the memories decreased until she was finally able to repeat the story with little emotion.

An Illustrative Case of Dissociative Reaction

Leahy and Martin (1967) describe a patient who was in his middle forties when first seen by the authors. Since returning from service in World War II he had been prone to episodes that involved altered states of consciousness. In these he would not recognize his wife, talk to her as though she were French, speak of prisoners of war, and walk around the house brandishing a knife. On several occasions a doctor had been called and had given him a sedative. He had no memory of the episodes afterwards. There was nothing unusual in the patient's childhood or family background and his marriage of 28 years had been relatively happy but for the disturbing episodes.

During an initial interview he could give no explanation for his unusual behavior, and there were no neurological indications of organic brain disorder. Under hypnosis, however, he told about an experience that had occurred 10 years previously. During World War II he found himself separated from his regular unit, with an officer unknown to him, and both of them in charge of four German prisoners. While stopping to rest in a small hut the officer, to the patient's horror, ordered him to shoot the unarmed prisoners. He refused to do this and in the ensuing argument threw his rifle to the officer, telling him to do the shooting. He then became afraid that the officer might shoot him, and in panic he crashed through the flimsy wall of the hut and ran back to his unit. While telling this story the patient became very emotional and seemed to relive the experience, including finally throwing himself against the wall with such force that he had to be restrained.

The hypnotic reexperiencing of the incident was repeated on several occasions and there seemed to be considerable improvement. Following discharge from the hospital he remained free of his amnesic episodes, however, for only a short period of time. He was finally readmitted to the hospital 10 years later with the episodes, if anything, even more severe. The patient was again asked to relive the original incident, but this time when he began to throw himself against the wall he was asked simply to tell the story without physically acting it out. After some initial resistance he described how after escaping from the hut he had run a few hundred yards but had then stopped, worried about the prisoners' fate. He returned, and meeting the officer alone outside the hut, had stabbed him to death with his bayonet. During the description he first expressed intense anger at the officer but then wept and expressed great sorrow at his action. Again the story was repeated on several subsequent occasions under hypnosis.

Eight months after discharge from the hospital the patient was completely free of the amnesic episodes. Previously the interval between episodes had never been longer than a week or two. A symptom that had persisted for 20 years had apparently been removed by reexperiencing the original traumatic incident. In contrast to the case of Kate Fox it was not possible in the present case to obtain independent evidence for the actual occurrence of the incident, although it seems reasonable to assume that something like it did occur.

Hysterical Personality

Many characteristics of the more extreme symptomatology seen in neurotic disorders are also seen in less extreme forms in individuals that would not be considered neurotic. This is not surprising if we view neurosis as simply an extreme point along a severity-of-handicap dimension. Thus, there are individuals with characteristic tendencies to be anxious, depressed and self-critical, or overly controlled and prone to compulsive rituals, but who are not handicapped enough by these traits to be considered neurotic. There does not seem to be any particular issue at stake here. In the case of hysterical personality, however, it seems that a certain pattern of personality traits is sometimes considered to represent a diagnostic category even though no conversion or dissociative reactions are present.

Chodoff and Lyons (1958) reviewed the literature and summarized seven characteristics of the hysterical personality on which there was general agreement: 1) self-centeredness, vanity; 2) exhibitionistic, overly dramatic; 3) emotionally labile, excitable; 4) emotional shallowness, affected; 5) sexualization of all relationships, sexually provocative; 6) sexually frigid in actual intercourse; 7) demanding, dependent. The authors then studied 17 patients with conversion reactions and reported that only three showed this pattern of traits. They concluded that although there are neurotic patients with this pattern of traits there is no close relationship between these traits and conversion reactions. This is probably too small a sample to be certain that there is no relationship, but it does suggest caution in assuming one. They further proposed that this particular pattern of traits suggests a caricature of the feminine role, given exaggerated importance as a diagnostic entity by *male* psychiatrists. If psychiatry had been dominated by female psychiatrists perhaps we would have a special diagnostic category based on an unflattering constellation of traits revolving around insecure masculinity. A common version of the hysterical personality involves a woman who seeks a dependent relationship with older, fatherly men. She snares such men with sexual provocativeness but is unable to relate to them in adult fashion, being more interested in gratifying childish dependency needs than in developing a mature sexual relationship. The relationship is likely to be mutually unsatisfactory and may not last long. The neurotic quality of the problem may be further indicated by a tendency to become involved in a succession of such unhappy relationships without learning from experience.

DEPRESSIVE REACTION

In practice it is not always easy to make a sharp distinction between neurotic depressions and psychotic depressions. We may be dealing only with a dimension of severity from normal to neurotic to psychotic, or there may be separate disorders with distinctive causative factors. The question remains unresolved. A depressive reaction is likely to be labeled neurotic, however, if there are environmental circumstances that played an important role in its precipitation, and the symptoms are only moderately severe and do not include delusional distortions of reality. Neurotic depression is sometimes referred to as reactive depression in accord with the assumed importance of situational factors.

The symptom picture itself can be characterized as an extension of the normal grief reaction with strong self-depreciatory tendencies. Thus the individual reports feelings of sadness, despondency and discouragement; may have crying spells; loses interest in his job, recreation, friends, and family; becomes slowed down in speech and physical activity; does not sleep well at night; loses his appetite; may be somewhat agitated and irritable; worries about his physical health. Thoughts of suicide and actual attempts at suicide may occur but are less likely than in the psychotic level depression.

The neurotic depressive reaction is frequently precipitated by a loss such as the death of a parent, spouse, close friend, or child; or the severance of a relationship by a boyfriend, girlfriend, or spouse; or a failure in school or at work, which usually has implications in terms of interpersonal rejection. These events are likely to make anyone feel depressed. The difference for the neurotic is that his depression is more severe, and it does not go away in a reasonable period of time—he cannot shake it off.

REFERENCES

Breuer, J., & Freud, S. Studies in hysteria. *The complete works of Sigmund Freud.* London: Hogarth Press, 1953.

Cameron, N. *Personality development and psychopathology: A dynamic approach.* Boston: Houghton Mifflin, 1963.

Carter, J. W. A case of reactional dissociation. *Amer. J. Orthopsychiat.,* 1937, **7,** 219–224.

Chodoff, P., & Lyons, H. Hysteria, the hysterical personality and "hysterical" conversion. *Amer. J. Psychiat.,* 1958, **114,** 734–740.

Lader, M. H. Palmer skin conductance measures in anxiety and phobic states. *J. psychosom. Res.*, 1967, **11**, 271–281.

Leahy, M. R., & Martin, I. C. A. Successful hypnotic abreaction after twenty years. *Brit. J. Psychiat.*, 1967, **113**, 383–385.

Leonard, W. E. *The locomotive God.* New York: Appleton-Century-Crofts, 1927.

CHAPTER THREE

ANXIETY AND OTHER EMOTIONS

It is self-evident that emotional reactions are intimately involved in neurotic processes, as indicated by the common use of such terms as "emotionally disturbed" as synonymous with neurotic disorder. Studies of emotion in man and other animals, however, have been distinguished by lack of general agreement as to what emotion is and how one measures it. In view of the close and perhaps central relationship of emotion to neurotic disorder it is important to consider the concept of emotion and its measurable manifestations in some detail.

The presence of an emotional reaction is inferred from three sources: self-reports about subjective experience; motoric behavior; and physiological responses. We might, for example, conclude that a person is having an emotional reaction of anger if he says "I hate you"; if he clenches his fists and stares fixedly at you; and if his blood pressure increases. Unfortunately, the definition and measurement of emotional reactions is not always this simple. The three sources of measurement do not always agree, and other kinds of psychological functions that might best be labeled motivational or cognitive are not readily distinguishable from those labeled emotional. In this chapter we shall see to what extent self-report, behavioral, and physiological responses permit us to distinguish emotional states thought to be especially relevant to neurotic disorders. We shall emphasize anxiety and grief, and consider briefly anger, shame, disgust, and certain positive emotions.

ANXIETY OR FEAR

An extremely fearful person is likely to report subjective experiences of apprehension, impending danger, tension, inability to concentrate, going to pieces, and a wish to flee or escape; behaviorally he may run away from or otherwise avoid his immediate situation, be generally disorganized with resulting impairment in speech, motor coordination, and in the performance of complex problem solving tasks; and physiologically show responses largely mediated by the autonomic nervous system. A more detailed consideration of physiological responses will be given in a later section.

It is important to distinguish between stimulus-oriented and response-oriented definitions of anxiety. A stimulus orientation defines anxiety in terms of the circumstances (external situations or internal thoughts) that elicit anxiety, and a response orientation defines anxiety in terms of the responses that compose the anxiety reaction. A distinction, for example, between anxiety about being castrated (a central concept in psychoanalytic theory) and anxiety about being rejected by or separated from the mother would seem to be in terms of what the person is afraid of, that is, the stimulus, rather than in terms of a difference in the anxiety response itself. The usual distinction between fear as reality based and anxiety as irrational also refers primarily to whether the eliciting stimulus involves a real danger rather than a difference in response. I shall emphasize a response-oriented definition, and take the position that, until shown otherwise, the anxiety response is the same regardless of the stimulus. Thus the terms fear and anxiety are considered synonymous unless explicitly stated otherwise.

Novelty or strangeness has been proposed as an unlearned elicitor of fear in many animal species. Hebb (1946), for example, reported that novel stimuli such as an anesthetized chimpanzee, a skull, and a clay model of a chimpanzee head would create terror in chimpanzees. Hebb suggested that an animal had to have prior visual experience with some object in the environments so that these objects could become familiar and thereby provide the necessary contrast for novel objects. The human infant does not show the well-known fear or distress reaction to strangers until about 6 to 8 months of age, presumably because he must first come to clearly recognize the familiar face of his mother before strangeness can be perceived.

Not all novel stimuli have the same power to elicit fear responses, however, and there is evidence that certain stimuli always elicit a fear response in some animal species. Sackett (1966) has shown that the picture of a "threatening" monkey, a characteristic facial expression involving baring of the teeth and a direct gaze, reliably elicits fear behavior in infant monkeys between 2 to 4 months of age, but not before that age. These monkeys had been reared in visual isolation from birth so that there was no opportunity to learn a connection between the visual threat stimulus and fear. Innate maturational processes would seem to be involved.

As one moves from the "lower" animals to man, most behavior patterns become more modifiable by learning and less tied to unlearned eliciting stimuli. Nevertheless there may be residual tendencies inherited from our primate ancestors that make us prone to be somewhat more fearful of certain stimuli than others, for example, novel stimuli at certain stages of development or the mutilated human body.

PHYSIOLOGICAL RESPONSES AND ANXIETY

It is important to understand the physiological aspects of the anxiety reaction not only as an aid to general comprehension of the nature of neurotic disorders but also because physiological measures are likely to be useful in assessing improvement with treatment and in monitoring the treatment process.

The Autonomic Nervous System

Many physiological responses associated with anxiety occur in the autonomic nervous system. This system primarily regulates the internal environment involving such processes as digestion, elimination, and blood pressure, and is composed of two divisions, the sympathetic and the parasympathetic. The center most importantly involved in activating and integrating the autonomic divisions is the hypothalamus. The posterior part of the hypothalamus primarily activates the sympathetic division and the anterior part of the hypothalamus primarily activates the parasympathetic division.

Sympathetic division. Arousal of this division helps an organism cope with emergency situations by "flight or fight" or other reactions involving the expenditure of unusual effort (Cannon, 1929). The biological significance of most sympathetic reactions is reasonably clear. The rate and force of contraction of the heart increase, and blood vessels to the viscera (stomach, intestines, and colon) and skin constrict so that the blood supply to the heart, the muscles, and the brain is increased. The combination of increased cardiac output and constriction of visceral and skin blood vessels results in an increase in blood pressure. Salivation in the mouth, muscular contractions in the stomach and intestines, and gastric secretions are inhibited. Bronchial passages in the lungs are dilated to permit greater oxygen intake to meet higher rates of body metabolism. The pupils dilate to increase visual sensitivity, and sweating occurs on the palmar surfaces of the hands and feet.

The adrenal medulla gland is stimulated to secrete epinephrine and norepinephrine into the blood stream.[1] Epinephrine tends to sustain many of the sympathetic reactions initiated directly by sympathetic nerves. For example, it acts directly on the heart to increase the rate and force of contraction and, by action in certain brain centers, may maintain a general sympathetic nervous system response. Epinephrine also produces certain effects not otherwise caused by direct neural stimulation. One of the more important effects of this kind is to cause the liver to convert glycogen to glucose (blood sugar) to provide additional metabolic fuel.

Circulating norepinephrine produces constriction of the blood vessels in the skin and viscera. Norepinephrine is also secreted by the adrenal medulla, but in addition is the substance that plays a part in the chemical transmission of nerve impulses from the end of sympathetic nerves to the smooth muscles of the viscera and blood vessels. Most of the norepinephrine circulating in the blood and found in the urine is probably produced at these sympathetic nerve endings rather than by the adrenal medulla.

Parasympathetic division. This division functions to conserve rather than expend bodily resources. Thus activation results in heart rate decrease and dilation of skin and visceral blood vessels. The accompanying drop in blood pressure tends to decrease the utilization of fuels throughout the body. Parasympathetic stimulation promotes digestive processes including increased muscle activity and dilation of blood vessels in the stomach and intestinal tracts, and increased secretion of gastric juices in the stomach. Eliminative processes are also facilitated. The pupil is constricted to reduce external stimulation.

Reciprocal inhibition. Reciprocal inhibition means that facilitating and inhibiting neurons connected to the same muscle group are also interconnected in such a way at spinal or higher levels of the central nervous system so that activation of one type of neuron inhibits the activation of the other type. When, for example, the posterior hypothalamus is stimulated to produce sympathetic activation, the anterior hypothalamus is inhibited to reduce parasympathetic activation, and vice versa. The result of this reciprocal inhibition is to amplify the effects of the system being activated since many functions such as heart rate are affected in opposite ways by sympathetic and parasympathetic stimulation.

---

[1] The terms adrenaline and noradrenaline are synonymous with epinephrine and norepinephrine, respectively.

Homeostasis and habituation. Homeostasis is a general term refer-ring to a state of equilibrium in a dynamic system. The autonomic system plays a role in maintaining certain balances within the body, for example, in maintaining body temperature within certain limits. More relevant to our concerns are attempts to restore equilibrium after psychologically produced imbalances have occurred. Thus, after sympathetic activation has resulted in increased blood pressure, pressure sensitive receptors in the aorta and other arteries send neural impulses to certain brain centers, which in turn cause blood vessel dilation and heart rate decrease. The re-sult is a drop in blood pressure. Homeostasis is achieved through sys-tems of this kind in which forces are set in operation by the original re-sponse that tend to dampen or reverse that response. The principle is the same as for the thermostat that regulates the temperature level of a house. Reciprocal inhibition works in an opposite fashion; forces are set in mo-tion by the original response that tend to further increase or amplify that response. Such a system, if allowed to go unchecked, would destroy equi-librium or homeostasis. In the well-functioning autonomic system the ini-tial amplifying effects of reciprocal inhibition are eventually reversed by homeostatic controls. If a series of arousing stimuli separated by intervals of no stimulation are presented to an organism, autonomic responses char-acteristically show a progressive decrease in magnitude. This process is called *habituation.*

Individual differences in autonomic response. Individuals vary widely in their characteristic autonomic responses to stress (Lacey, Bate-man, & Van Lehn, 1953; Engel, 1960). For example, some respond with large heart rate and blood pressure responses and show little change in palmar sweating; others show the reverse. Richmond and Lustman (1955) report stable individual differences in autonomic response even in the young infant, suggesting the possibility of hereditary influences. Individual differences in general level of autonomic reactivity as well as in specific patterns of response may well have implications for the development of certain autonomic correlates of anxiety.

Pituitary Adrenocortical System

One aspect of the endocrine system that is intimately involved in emo-tional reactions to both physical and psychological stress is the pituitary–adrenocortical system. When the posterior hypothalamus is acti-vated in response to physical or psychological stress, in addition to pro-ducing a general sympathetic response, it releases hormones which stimulate the nearby pituitary gland to secrete adrenocorticotrophic hormone (ACTH) into the blood stream. This hormone in turn causes the adrenal cortex gland to secrete adrenocortical hormones (ACH) which generally aid the organism in responding to stress. The adrenocortical hormones and the results of their metabolism can be measured from samples of blood, blood plasma, or urine. The pituitary–adrenocortical system seems to be responsive to almost any severe and/or chronic stress, either physical or psychological, and does not seem to show distinctive features associated with different emotional reactions.

Physiological Responses in Patients with Anxiety Reactions

Strong sympathetic arousal is frequently indicated by rapid or irregular heart rate and breathing, increased systolic blood pressure, dryness in the mouth resulting from inhibited salivation, sweating on the palmar surfaces of the hands and feet, coldness in the extremities, shivering, and muscular tremor. Parasympathetic involvement is reflected in such symptoms as stomach distress, diarrhea, and increased frequency of urination.

A variation that may occur in acute conditions is fainting. The physiological component in the fainting response, in contrast to the mixed sympathetic-parasympathetic pattern just described, is largely parasympathetic in nature, involving abrupt dilation of the blood vessels in the viscera, slowing of the heart rate, drop in blood pressure, and loss of muscle tone. These effects result in a sharp decrease in the blood supply to the brain and produce loss of consciousness. The parasympathetic-dominated fainting response is likely to occur only in strong, acute fear.

The first and more common pattern, involving both autonomic divisions but usually with a sympathetic emphasis, can occur as either a chronic or acute reaction. Gellhorn (1967) has suggested that in cases of pathological anxiety there is a failure in the reciprocally inhibiting mechanisms in the hypothalamic system, and strong arousal in one division overflows into the other, producing the mixed parasympathetic and sympathetic effects. In the following sections we will review research on levels of physiological arousal, habituation, and homeostatic control in anxiety patients.

High levels of arousal. Research generally indicates that patients diagnosed as having an anxiety reaction or otherwise selected for the prominence of anxiety symptoms show high levels of sympathetic and adrenocortical arousal. In making this generalization it is important to stress the necessity of selecting a patient group where anxiety is the prominent symptom. Patients with mixed or other neurotic symptom pictures do not necessarily show unusual arousal.

Persky et al. (1959) measured blood plasma levels of adrenocortical hormones and urinary products of these hormones in a group of anxious patients and a control group of normals. Measures were obtained on a pre-experimental day, during which stressful aspects of the experience were minimized, and on three successive days during which the patients were made to fail on a simple perceptual task that involved no physical effort. On each day measures were obtained immediately before, immediately after, and four hours after the failure experience or at the equivalent time intervals on the pre-experimental day. Both indices of adrenocortical functioning in the anxious patients were elevated relative to the control group at all points throughout the sessions *including the pre-experimental day*. And this elevation was as high or higher on the pre-experimental day for the anxiety patients as on the succeeding "stress" days. Similar results were obtained for a second group of anxious patients subjected to a stressful interview procedure.

Persky et al. had initially expected the pre-experimental session to provide a nonstress baseline from which they could measure relative increases under stress. Instead, the unfamiliar laboratory situation with associated blood sampling and other tests and with unknown implications for their hospital treatment seems to have produced as much anxiety in the patients as the situations designed to be anxiety arousing. Two important conclusions can be drawn from this study: 1) the anxiety arousing qualities of a situation should not be too narrowly conceived by an investigator, and 2) anxious patients probably do manifest greater adrenocortical arousal than normals in a variety of situations.

This tendency for anxious patients to show anxiety arousal during prestress periods (sometimes called "basal," "rest," or "relaxation" periods) has been dramatically shown in studies by Kelly (1966) and Kelly and Walter (1968). These authors used a measure of forearm blood flow that appears to be especially sensitive to anxiety level, and they also provide comparisons among a number of diagnostic groups. Forearm blood flow is measured by a rather involved apparatus that encloses the forearm and is sensitive to volume changes. Blood circulation is temporarily stopped at one-minute intervals and the rate of increase in forearm volume is taken as an indication of rate of blood flow to the forearm muscles. Muscle accounts for about 59% of the total volume; bone and fat that have little blood supply account for 28%; and skin accounts for 13%. Dilation of blood vessels in forearm muscle, causing increased blood flow, is mediated largely by sympathetic nerves and to a lesser extent by circulating epinephrine. Measurement procedures and terminology associated with other autonomic responses used in this and other studies to be reviewed are described in Table 1.

Measures were obtained during a 15-minute "basal" period and during a brief period of stress where they were required to subtract numbers as rapidly as possible while being continually harassed and criticized. The results for forearm blood flow as well as heart rate and self-report anxiety ratings are shown in Table 2. The anxiety group had significantly higher blood flow rates during the "basal" period than did the normal controls.

TABLE 1: Measurement and Terminology Associated with Palmar Skin Resistance, Heart Rate, and Blood Pressure

PALMAR SKIN RESISTANCE

Instrumentation

Two electrodes are attached to palmar surfaces, usually of two fingers, and resistance to small current flow is measured. Sympathetic actuation of sweat glands causes drop in electrical resistance.

Galvanic Skin Response (GSR)

Discrete drop in resistance that occurs after an arousing stimulus. Resistance usually returns to near original value within 5 to 10 seconds. Can be measured as change in resistance, R, in ohms, or change in conductance, $C = \frac{1}{R}$.

Spontaneous or Nonspecific GSR's

Same as above except that no obvious eliciting stimulus is present. Uusually measured as frequency of occurrence of GSR's of certain magnitude within some specified time interval.

Level of Skin Resistance or Conductance

The average level of resistance or conductance during some specified time interval.

HEART RATE

Instrumentation

Electrodes are attached to body to pick up muscle action potentials associated with contraction of heart. Strongest signals are obtained from chest near heart.

Common Measures

The electrocardiogram (EKG) shows sharp spikes on a chart that are separated by the time interval between beats. This output can be converted by a cardiotachometer to provide a direct reading of heart rate in beats per minute. The average rate, the lowest rate and the highest rate during a specified time interval have all been used as measures.

BLOOD PRESSURE

Instrumentation

An inflatable cuff is attached to upper part of the arm and inflated until the pulse beat cannot be heard in a stethoscope placed below cuff. The air is gradually let out of cuff. The air pressure at the point where the pulse beat is first heard again is called systolic blood pressure. As the air is continued to be let out of the cuff a point is reached where the pulse beat is again no longer heard. The air pressure corresponding to this point is called diastolic blood pressure. The instrument used in these measurements is called a *sphygmomanometer*. It is possible to automate this procedure so that blood pressure readings can be taken at regular time intervals and recorded on chart paper.

Common Measures

If a near continuous measure is not obtained automatically it is desirable to use an average of several readings because of the unreliability of a single reading. The units of measurement are mm of mercury corresponding to air pressure at the systolic and diastolic points.

During stress both groups increased with the normals increasing more, so that the stress measures were not significantly different.

TABLE 2: Forearm Blood Flow, Heart Rate, and Anxiety Self Rating for Different Diagnostic Categories[a]

	N	Basal			Stress		
		Blood Flow (ml/100 ml/ min.)	Heart Rate	Self Rating	Blood Flow (ml/100 ml/ min.)	Heart Rate	Self Rating
Chronic anxiety	41	4.45	97.34	3.98	7.69	110.37	6.51
Agitated depression	15	3.54	89.20	4.87	5.46	98.27	6.73
Schizophrenia	20	3.31	88.30	4.44	5.47	96.20	5.67
Obsessional neurosis	20	2.65	85.80	3.80	6.38	102.30	7.45
Phobic state	32	2.26	85.88	3.06	5.22	99.16	5.63
Hysteria	9	2.20	82.33	2.56	4.68	94.00	4.89
Non-agitated depression	43	2.13	86.42	3.55	4.78	98.88	6.43
Personality disorder	15	1.90	76.40	3.40	5.21	90.93	6.60
Depersonalization	8	1.84	88.25	4.25	4.94	100.50	5.88
Normal control	60	2.21	73.72	1.64	8.26	97.88	5.02

[a] Adapted from a table presented by Kelly and Walter (1968).

The measures of blood flow, heart rate, and self-ratings of anxiety for other diagnostic groups, especially the obsessional, phobic, and hysterical reactions, are of interest. Note that for all three of these groups basal and stress measures are less than for the anxiety group, a finding consistent with clinical observations of lower general anxiety levels in these groups.

Anxious patients, then, do not appear to be very discriminating in terms of the situations in which they respond with anxiety. Normals on the other hand show anxiety arousal in circumstances where one might expect some degree of arousal but do not show it in other situations.

Higher levels of arousal for anxiety reaction patients have been found using other measures: systolic blood pressure (Malmo & Shagass, 1952); muscle tension (Davis, Malmo, & Shagass, 1954; Sainsbury, 1964); palmar skin conductance levels (Lader & Wing, 1964). Shagass and Jones (1957) found that anxiety reaction patients had to receive higher doses of a sedative to achieve a given criterion of drowsiness than did normals or other neurotic patients. Similarly, the research indicating greater facilitation of GSR conditioning (Beam, 1955; Bitterman & Holtzman, 1952; Welsh & Kubis, 1947) or eyeblink conditioning (Franks, 1956; Spence, 1964) in groups assessed to be highly anxious indicates a higher level of general arousal. It is important to point out that the conditioning studies referred to used simple and easy learning tasks. Highly anxious subjects are likely to be inferior in learning complex or difficult tasks. The simple conditioning superiority may, in fact, reflect a general *sensitization* to all stimuli rather than a specific learned association.

Another finding that demonstrates the high susceptibility to arousal of anxiety patients is the tendency for injected epinephrine to produce a full-fledged anxiety attack; similar injections in normal controls produce milder effects of much shorter duration. Associated subjective experiences such as apprehension are much less severe in normals. Tomkins, Sturgis, and Wearn (1919) report results of this kind.

Along similar lines, Pitts and McClure (1967) report that lactic acid infusion produced acute anxiety attacks with prolonged aftereffects in anxiety patients but only temporary and limited physiological reactions confined largely to paresthesia (tingling or other sensations in certain parts of the body) and "shakiness" in normal controls. They conclude that the lactate ion plays an important role in the anxiety reaction, and cite other studies (Cohen & White, 1950; Jones & Mellersh, 1946) that found no differences in blood lactic acid levels during rest but a significantly greater rise during work or exercise for anxiety patients than normals. Pitts and McClure had also, in counterbalanced order with the same subjects, infused a mixture of lactic acid and calcium chloride during one session, and a placebo of glucose in saline solution in another session. The calcium chloride greatly reduced the magnitude and duration of the anxiety reaction, especially for the anxious patients; and neither anxiety patients nor normals showed much response to the glucose infusions. Low blood calcium levels are known to produce some of the physiological symptoms associated with anxiety, and the authors proposed the following theory: epinephrine release in anxiety patients produces unusual amounts of lactic acid which in turn somehow inhibits calcium metabolism. The resulting low level of calcium in the blood is thought to cause the anxiety reaction. Their speculations deserve careful study, but on the basis of their results alone one can only conclude that above-normal amounts of lactic acid seem to produce some anxiety-like physiological responses.

It is possible that lactic acid or epinephrine produce only certain limited features of the physiological responses associated with anxiety, and that on the basis of past conditioning processes (discussed in Chapter 5) these partial responses elicit the full-scale anxiety reaction. The subject's cognitive interpretation of the initial response as portending the dreaded attack may also facilitate the vicious circle.

Habituation. To measure habituation one must present subjects with a series of discrete arousal-stimuli with sufficiently long intervals between stimuli so that considerable recovery can occur. The intervals may be of the order of minutes, hours, or days. Most experimental research to date has studied habituation within the confines of one session using relatively short intervals of about a minute.

Davis, Malmo, and Shagass (1954) report habituation data to a series of 10 startle stimuli given at one minute intervals. Increase in muscular tension in the forearm to each stimulus was recorded, and the anxiety patients were found to be slower in habituating (the authors use the term *adaptation*). Malmo, Shagass, and Heslam (1951) report a similar finding for systolic blood pressure, that is, anxiety patients continued to show greater increases in blood pressure to repeated brief stresses than normals.

Lader and Wing (1964) and Lader (1967) report studies of habituation of the galvanic skin response (GSR) that are noteworthy for the careful selection of "pure" anxiety or phobic patient groups. In both studies subjects were given 20 presentations of a 1000-cps tone at varying intervals.

Skin conductance results for the Lader and Wing study are shown in Figure 1. The 20 anxiety patients started at a higher level in "rest" and showed a slight rise throughout the session while the 20 normals showed an overall drop. The rise at point 14 for both groups reflects the beginning of the tone series. The average GSR's to the successive tones are shown in Figure 2. There was no overall difference in magnitude of GSR between the two groups. In fact for the first five tones the normals gave larger GSR's than the anxiety patients. These larger GSR's for the normals may

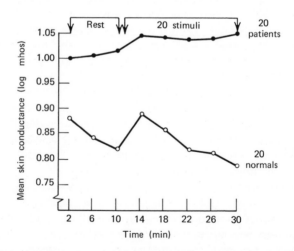

FIGURE 1.   The effects of 20 auditory stimuli on the skin conductances. Each point represents the mean of four log conductance readings (Lader & Wing, 1964).

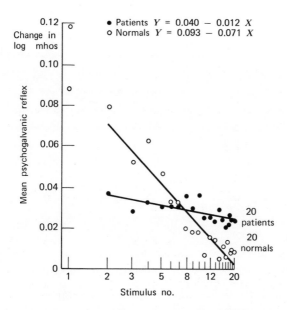

FIGURE 2. Habituation regression lines of the psychogalvanic reflex (Lader & Wing, 1964).

reflect the fact that the normals' pretone levels of conductance are much lower than the anxiety patients', as shown in Figure 1. There is considerable evidence that change in many autonomic responses will be greater if they start from low initial levels. The interesting aspect of the data in Figure 2 is the greater rate of habituation for the normals as indicated by the different slopes of the lines fitted to the data of the two groups. The GSR to the first tone was omitted in fitting these straight lines. Lader and Wing showed statistically that the average rate of habituation was significantly less for the anxiety patients.

Figure 3 (p. 32) shows results for spontaneous GSR's, those occurring during the 40-second period before each tone. The anxiety patients showed a significantly higher level, but there was no difference in rate of decrease in this measure over the session.

Lader (1967) repeated this procedure on different groups of 16 anxiety patients and 75 normals, but also included groups of 18 anxiety-with-depression patients, 19 agoraphobics (those with fear of open spaces, forms of transportation, elevators, and shops), 18 social phobics (fear of eating in public, attending public gatherings, speaking in public, and conversations with strangers), and 19 specific phobics (fear of spiders, birds, dogs,

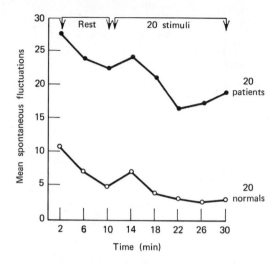

FIGURE 3. The effects of 20 auditory stimuli on the number of spontaneous skin conductance fluctuations. Each point represents the mean number of fluctuations counted for four periods of 40 seconds (Lader & Wing, 1964).

cats, etc.). The results for the comparisons between the anxiety and normal groups were essentially the same as in the previous study and provide further confirmation of those findings. The results for the other groups are of interest in that they provide objective evidence for the varying degrees of pervasiveness of the anxiety reaction found in these groups. Numbers reflecting the average rate of habituation (statistically corrected for differences in initial GSR magnitude) for the various groups are as follows: anxiety-with-depression, 22; anxiety reaction, 29; agoraphobia, 39; social phobia, 39; specific phobia, 68; and normals, 72.

Similar findings were obtained for the average number of spontaneous GSR's obtained over the whole session: anxiety-with-depression, 37; anxiety reaction, 36; agoraphobia, 32; social phobia, 33; specific phobia, 15; and normals, 8. For both habituation and spontaneous GSR's, statistical analyses indicated overall significant differences among groups. Subsequent tests showed that only the specific phobics and normals were significantly different on both measures from all other groups.

These results further support the idea that the specific phobics, whose fear frequently involves animals, are indeed not anxious except in the phobic situation. Individuals whose phobias involved social stimuli showed some degree of anxiety arousal in this experimental situation and fell between the anxiety-reaction group and the specific phobics. The anxiety-with-depression group was indistinguishable from the anxiety group. This finding suggests that the anxiety-depression symptoms were relatively general, and the effects of anxiety and depression were not incompatible, or, at least, that they alternated closely in time.

Homeostatic control. Homeostatic processes can be measured in various ways; for example, by measuring speed of return to a pre-arousal level after termination of a brief arousing stimulus or during a continuing stressful experience.

Malmo, Shagass, and Davis (1950) and Davis, Malmo, and Shagass (1954) report two studies in which anxiety patients showed slower recovery than normal controls from a startle response induced by a loud noise. The second study was referred to previously with respect to the habituation findings, and the results from this same study relevant to recovery rates are shown in Figure 4. Anxiety patients showed somewhat higher muscle tension levels prior to and in response to stimulation. Especially striking is the slower recovery rate of the anxious patients. It is of some interest that the muscle tension response and recovery occur within one second, a much shorter time interval than is involved in autonomic response and recovery.

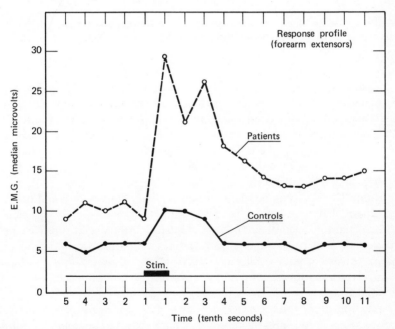

FIGURE 4. Comparison of patients and controls in forearm muscle potential amplitude for each tenth-second preceding and following stimulation. Each point on the curve is based on the averaged data from the first four stimulations (Davis, Malmo, & Shagass, 1954).

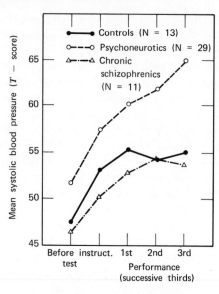

Mirror drawing test (circle)

FIGURE 5.   Mean blood pressure during mirror drawing test (circle). Note continuous rise in curve for psychoneurotics (Malmo & Shagass, 1952).

Malmo and Shagass (1952) administered a stressful mirror-drawing test to normal controls, anxiety patients, and chronic schizophrenics. The results for systolic blood pressure are shown in Figure 5. The anxiety patients again start at a somewhat higher level, but the finding relevant to our present concern is the lack of any tendency to adapt during successive thirds of the stressful task in contrast to both normal and schizophrenic patients. Similar results were found for heart rates.

Rubin (1964) obtained measures of pupillary constriction and dilation, and found that a group of neurotic patients (not especially selected in terms of the presence of anxiety) responded to stress with alternations of sympathetic and parasympathetic responses that were slow to recover, a finding consistent with Gellhorn's (1967) proposal that pathological anxiety involves a malfunctioning of the reciprocal inhibition mechanism in the hypothalamus.

Physiological responses in anxiety reactions: Conclusions. Groups selected to represent relatively "pure" cases of anxiety reaction are likely to show greater physiological arousal to stress, slower habituation to repeated stresses, and slower recovery from stress. These findings should not be altogether surprising, since informal observations of or self-reports about physiological arousal frequently contribute to the diagnostic process that results in the label anxiety reaction. These studies, however, provide objective confirmation for clinically based assumptions about the general role of physiological responses in anxiety reactions; more important, they permit us to take a closer look at processes such as habituation and homeostatic control that may suggest new theories about the nature of the mechanisms involved.

The greater physiological response of anxiety patients to stress is perhaps the least clear-cut finding. Some inconsistency in previous research on this point may reflect the tendency of anxiety patients to already be physiologically aroused during so-called rest or prestress periods with accordingly little room for further increase during stress. Arousal during rest periods is consistent with the idea that anxiety patients respond with anxiety in many situations. This lack of discrimination in response may reflect anxiety conditioning or generalization to many stimuli in the external environment, or it may be mediated by internal thought stimuli in which the person "makes himself anxious" by imagining various unfortunate things that might happen, or some combination of all these factors. The greater number of spontaneous GSR's found in anxiety patients suggests the importance of internal thoughts since there are no external stimuli correlated with their occurrence. Or a highly aroused physiological system may, indeed, show spontaneous GSR's without external or internal eliciting stimuli.

There is no inevitable reason why a tendency toward overarousal should be accompanied by a lack of normal habituation. It would seem possible for a group of individuals to show unusually high levels of arousal to all stimuli but to habituate at a normal or ever faster than normal rate. The evidence seems to suggest, however, that anxiety patients show both higher levels of arousal *and* slower habituation. In normal habituation certain inhibitory mechanisms must operate that reduce the organism's response to repeated presentations of the *same* stimulus. The slow habituation of anxiety patients suggests that there is something defective in these inhibitory mechanisms.

There also appears to be something defective in the homeostatic recovery capacities of the anxiety patient. Malmo (1966) has suggested that the mechanisms responsible for slow homeostatic recovery is a defect in the inhibitory functions of the descending brain-stem reticular system. In normal functioning, when arousal at higher brain levels reaches a certain magnitude, impulses going down the descending pathways activate the inhibitory centers, which in turn inhibit the arousal centers—thus promoting a return to prearousal levels.

Although neurophysiological speculations may suggest researchable ideas, it is beyond the scope of this book to consider them in detail. The complexities of the central nervous system are such that there are many possible mechanisms, including pathologically intense arousal processes as well as impaired inhibitory ones, that could account for the observed findings.

Patterns of Autonomic Response in Fear and Anger

Autonomic responses are associated with such processes as "orienting" to novel stimuli; physical effort; water, food, and sleep deprivation; sexual arousal; intense physical stimulation such as electric shock or loud noise; mental effort such as mental arithmetic; *and* emotions such as fear, anger, grief, and laughter. It is unlikely that measures of autonomic response will show distinctive patterns associated with each of these processes.

Some degree of differential response may occur, however. For example, heart rate decrease is a common immediate response to any novel stimulus that is not noxious. This may be part of a more general orienting response, that is, a kind of "what is it" response in which the organism appraises some new event in its environment. On the other hand sudden, intense stimuli are more likely to cause heart rate increase as part of a startle response or general defensive reaction against noxious stimulation.

Several studies have attempted to identify distinctive autonomic patterns associated with fear and anger. In some early work along these lines Ax (1953) and Schachter (1957) contrasted various autonomic measures obtained under experimental conditions aimed at inducing either a fear or an anger reaction. Funkenstein et al. (1957) likewise attempted to differentiate cardiovascular responses associated with fear and anger. In the latter study all subjects were given the same failure experience and subsequently assigned on the basis of an interview to various groups, including a group that directed anger outwardly and a group that responded with anxiety. The results for the specific autonomic measures were not completely consistent in these three studies, but the investigators suggested that autonomic responses associated with fear were similar to those produced by infused epinephrine, and those produced by anger were similar to those produced by infused norepinephrine. There were tendencies in these studies for diastolic blood pressure to increase in anger but *decrease* in fear. Heart rate increased in both but somewhat more in fear than anger. Estimations of cardiac output (blood volume per unit of time) were found to increase in fear but remain about the same or decrease in anger, and indices of peripheral vascular resistance (an indication of blood vessel constriction) were found to decrease in fear and increase in anger.

These early studies should be considered as only suggestive, because there are many methodological problems in research of this kind. For example, general intensity of arousal should be approximately the same for the experimental conditions, and independent behavioral and self-report evidence should be obtained to verify the appropriate designation of fear and anger to the arousal states.

Epinephrine and Norepinephrine in Fear and Anger

The suggestive trends in the above studies may be clarified if we look more closely at the functions of epinephrine and norepinephrine, and at the results of more recent studies relating fear and anger to these hormones.

Infusion studies. An obvious strategy for studying the relationship of hormones to emotion is to inject the hormone into subjects and measure its effects. In general, the physiological effects of infused epinephrine produce many of the effects of direct sympathetic neural stimulation. The effects of infused norepinephrine seem to be largely restricted to blood vessel constriction in the skin and viscera. Distinctive trends in response to epinephrine and norepinephrine can be seen most clearly in the patterns of cardiovascular responses as shown in Table 3.

The behavioral and self-report effects of epinephrine and norepinephrine are not as consistent as the physiological effects. With epi-

TABLE 3: Effects of Infused Epinephrine and Norepinephrine on Certain Cardiovascular Functions

Cardiovascular Function	Epinephrine	Norepinephrine
Heart rate	increase	little change
Systolic B.P.	increase	increase
Diastolic B.P.	little change or decrease	increase
Cardiac output	increase	little change
Blood flow to skeletal muscles	increase	little change
Blood flow to skin and viscera	little change	decrease
Peripheral resistance (reflects blood vessel constriction in skeletal muscles as well as skin and viscera)	decrease	increase

Note: These are general trends and there are, of course, individual differences in all these responses.

nephrine infusion subjects frequently report the subjective counterpart of the objectively measured physiological responses, that is, pounding of the heart in the chest and head, dryness of mouth, dizziness, and coldness in the extremities. They also occasionally report subjective experiences of apprehension, restlessness, and feelings of unreality. As will be shown in Chapter 6, however, self-report and behavioral manifestation can be greatly influenced by the subject's cognitive expectations and the social situation in which the infusions are given. Norepinephrine does not seem to produce consistent subjective experiences and sometimes produces no subjective experience at all (Frankenhaeuser, Jarpe, & Matell, 1960).

Secretion studies. Another research strategy is to arouse fear or anger experimentally, or by the selection of real life situations, and measure the urinary secretion of these hormones. Studies have not yielded consistent results. This lack of consistency probably results from the fact that there are such large individual differences in people's psychophysiological responses to the *same* arousing situation. Studies in which subjects given the same arousing "stress" are subsequently divided into fear and anger groups on the basis of behavioral and self-report measures obtained during or immediately after the stress have provided more consistent results.

Silverman and Cohen (1960) used a *g* tolerance test in which subjects are rotated on a large centrifuge until the centrifugal forces produce blackout. Silverman and Cohen thought that this measure might be especially sensitive to epinephrine-norepinephrine proportions because epinephrine tends to be associated with dilation of blood vessels in the muscles with a resulting pooling of blood in the muscular extremities and reduction of blood supply to the brain and eyes. High proportions of norepinephrine, with its strong blood vessel constricting effects in the skin and viscera, maintain an adequate supply of blood to the brain and eyes for a longer period of time during increasing centrifugal force. Thus subjects with high epinephrine proportions should black out with less *g* force than those with high norepinephrine proportions.

In their first experiment Silverman and Cohen found that subjects who scored high on an aggressiveness measure (based on stories told to pictures) had higher *g* tolerance than subjects who scored high on a passive-submissive measure. This is only indirect evidence for the role of epinephrine and norepinephrine; these physiological measures were not obtained.

In their second experiment they measured urinary epinephrine and norepinephrine before and immediately after the *g* tolerance test. The subjects were also provoked by arbitrary criticism at the beginning of the centrifuge test. Immediately after the test they were interviewed by a psychiatrist, who was not aware of *g* tolerance or hormone results, and were rated in terms of aggressive versus anxious reactions. The results of this study are summarized in Table 4.

It is clear that g tolerance increases with decreasing amounts of epinephrine and increasing amounts of norepinephrine. Furthermore, the trends are the same for measures of the hormones taken immediately before the test as for those taken after the test. Since the norepinephrine levels for high-g subjects were higher *before* the tolerance test, the possibility that the greater physical stress experienced by the high-g subjects could have produced the higher norepinephrine levels cannot be an explanation for the results. The relative proportion of epinephrine to norepinephrine is probably more highly related to g tolerance than the absolute amounts of epinephrine and norepinephrine considered separately.

TABLE 4: Psychophysiological Relationships in Centrifuge Stress[a]

| Subject | Black-Out Level (g) | Urinary Epinephrine and Norepinephrine (mgm/hr) | | | | Affect State by Interview Rating | |
| | | Control | | Stress | | | |
		Epin.	Norepin.	Epin.	Norepin.	Aggression	Anxiety
1	3.1 (low tolerance)	1.42	2.31	4.2	5.5	0	+ + +
2	3.3 (low tolerance)	1.22	1.64	3.9	5.7	+	+ + +
3	3.6 (average)	2.28	2.40	3.5	6.5	+ +	+ + +
4	3.9 (high average)	.66	2.66	2.73	9.9	+ + +	+ +
5	4.4 (high)	.99	2.96	3.5	9.9	+ + +	+
6	4.6+ (high)	.66	6.05	2.96	16.12	+ + +	0

[a] Adapted from a table provided by Silverman and Cohen (1960).

The right-hand columns of Table 4 include results based on the psychiatrist's 4-point rating scales of aggression and anxiety, ranging in intensity from 0 to + + +. High ratings on anxiety are associated with subjects who had low g tolerance, high amounts of epinephrine, and low amounts of norepinephrine. The reverse was true for subjects rated high on aggression. In a third experiment Silverman and Cohen used somewhat different procedures, and found similar results.

The relation between personality traits of aggressiveness and anxiousness and epinephrine–norepinephrine ratios suggested by Silverman and Cohen's first experiment has not been found consistently by other investigators, probably because of problems of validity of trait measurement and the variation from situation to situation of personality trait expression. Results similar to those of their second and third experiments have been found by other investigators. For example, Elmadjian, Hope, and Lamson (1957) found larger increases in norepinephrine than in epinephrine for hockey players during active competition and in psychiatric patients showing aggressive emotional outbursts. Larger increases in epinephrine were found for hockey players who observed but did not participate in the game and in psychiatric patients during staff conferences.

The importance of assessing the emotional reaction in the situation in which the hormone measures are taken should be emphasized again. Silverman and Cohen (1960), for example, describe a subject who experienced the centrifuge g tolerance test on one occasion and a stress involving criticism and electric shock on another occasion. On the g tolerance test he was rated high on anxiety, showed low g tolerance and had a high epinephrine–norepinephrine ratio. He responded with anger in the criticism and electric shock situation and showed a low epinephrine-norepinephrine ratio.

Although these studies suggest that circulating epinephrine-norepinephrine proportions are important correlates of the human fear and anger responses, it is possible that these hormones represent secondary features of arousal patterns and do not necessarily play a direct causative role in many aspects of the reaction. Gellhorn (1967), for example, provides evidence from animal experiments that suggests that prior hypothalamic balance toward the *parasympathetic* side is associated with anxiety and a high epinephrine-norepinephrine ratio. Conversely, prior hypothalamic sympathetic balance is associated with anger and low epinephrine-norepinephrine ratios. The exact mechanisms responsible for these relationships remain to be worked out, but the empirical evidence for a relationship between epinephrine-norepinephrine ratios and fear and anger is relatively strong at this time.

GRIEF

The emotion of grief is most commonly associated with the loss of some important source of need satisfaction (the term reinforcer will be used in Chapter 5). Individuals such as parents, spouse, or child become especially important as need satisfiers, and their loss or removal is especially potent in inducing grief. Bowlby (1960), Freud and Burlingham (1943), and Heinicke (1956) describe grief reactions that occurred in normal children 1 to 3 years of age when they were separated from their parents during wartime evacuation of London and during extended periods of hospitalization. First there is a period of protest during which the child cries a great deal, asks for his parents if he can talk, is restless, hyperactive, and easily angered. After about a week some children decrease these overt protests and manifest what has variously been called despair, depression, or withdrawal. They become unresponsive and lose interest in the environment. The facial muscles sag and the face presents the generally accepted features of sadness and dejection. Loud wailing and crying may be replaced with low-intensity whimpering or sobbing. Most children of this age are likely to recover after several weeks from this depression-withdrawal phase and return to a normal interest and responsiveness in their environment.

Adult grief is complicated by cultural influences and various learned inhibitions about grief expression. It nevertheless seems to follow in broad outline the same sequence as for the young child. Lindeman (1944) interviewed individuals who had lost close relatives in the Boston Coconut Grove fire, and Marris (1958) interviewed widows who had recently lost husbands. The initial reaction is frequently one of shock, disbelief, and an inability to accept the fact that the loss has occurred. The bereaved person may obsessively recall memories of incidents with the dead person, have a "sense" of the dead person's presence, or act as though the person still lived. Agitation, insomnia, lack of appetite, and reactions of irritation to reminders of the loss are common. Many features of this reaction are consistent with the notion that the person is "protesting" the loss.

As in the case for the young child, the period of protest is usually followed by a period of despair and depression-withdrawal. The person becomes apathetic and unresponsive, showing facial features of dejection. The more energetic wailing and crying that may have been present in the first phase gives way to occasional quiet sobbing as it did for the child. In time, however, the person begins to find new, and return to old, sources of need satisfaction and come back to a more or less normal life. This sequence is meant to represent a normal grief reaction to an important loss. The severity and duration vary markedly from person to person. Pathological or neurotic degrees of grief are associated with unusual severity and duration of the depression-withdrawal stage of the reaction.

Spitz (1945) has described severe and apparently irreversible states of physical retardation, psychological impairment, and withdrawal that accompanied the early placement of infants in a foundling home where very little individual attention and "mothering" was provided. Similar effects have been shown to occur in infant rhesus monkeys reared without contact with other monkeys (Harlow, 1958). The gross impairment associated with this early and continued lack of "mothering" undoubtedly encompasses more than just an extension of the emotional reaction of grief.

More relevant to an understanding of the extremes of the emotion of grief was a subsequent study by Spitz (1946) of infants of unwed mothers.

These infants were kept in a nursery and their mothers were encouraged to spend considerable time with them. From a sample of 123 infants observed during the first year of life, 19 were reported to have developed a clear-cut syndrome of depression. This reaction occurred only in infants whose mothers had to be away from them for about three months when the infants were some 6 to 10 months of age, but apparently did not occur in all such infants.

Initially the child was described as showing the facial expression of sadness but occasionally making some feeble attempt to respond to an observer and participate in play. He was likely to cling to the observer and react with "sorrowful disappointment" when the observer left. In the second stage the observer's approach provoked crying or screaming and little disappointment was shown on the observer's leaving. It happened that most of these depressive reactions were precipitated by their mother's leaving near the 6–8 month period during which most infants show a fear or distress reaction to strangers, and Spitz comments on the difference between the reaction of normal and depressed infants to strangers in this second stage. With the normal infant a stranger can overcome this fearful reaction within 2–10 minutes by simply remaining close with head averted and allowing the infant to take the initiative in establishing contact. With the depressed infants it would take up to an hour to achieve some kind of nonupsetting contact. In the final stages of the depressive reaction the outward appearance of the child was one of complete dejection. There was lack of responsiveness to environmental events, slowness of movement, general loss of muscle tone, refusal to eat and insomnia. The active weeping behavior of the second stage had given way to almost complete withdrawal and apathy.

The depressive reaction began about 4–6 weeks after the mother left and the availability of a substitute mother did not help much in most cases. There was no difference in the general stage of psychological and physical development prior to the mothers' leaving between the infants who became depressed and the infants whose mothers did not leave and who did not become depressed. The depressive reaction appeared to be reversible as indicated by the eventual return to normalcy of the infants when their mothers returned. Possible long-term effects of the separation, however, were not known.

In a more carefully conducted study Engel, Reichsman, and Segal (1956) report systematic observations of behavioral and physiological reactions in an infant girl who showed depressive reactions similar to the depression described by Spitz. The infant, Monica, was born with a defective esophagus which necessitated an operation a few days after birth to establish an opening for a tube into the stomach through which she could receive food. Until the age of five months, Monica seemed to progress normally; her parents had been living with her grandparents during this 'time, and apparently the grandmother had provided a lot of help. Monica's mother was generally uncomfortable about feeding her, and was afraid to fondle or hug her for fear of disturbing the tube. When Monica was five months old her parents moved away from the grandparents to an isolated farmhouse, and the mother became pregnant again. Monica started to become cranky and irritable, to cry all the time, and to lose weight. She was hospitalized for two extended periods of time during the next 18 months and showed improvement both times. This was especially true at the end of her second period of hospitalization, when an operation restored the normal use of her esophagus, an event accompanied by a marked improvement in the mother's attitude toward her.

For much of her hospitalization she was quite retarded for her age, being unable to sit up or speak at all. She did, however, develop positive relationships with some of the staff members, manifested by smiling, laughing, cooing, gurgling, and other signs of responsiveness. She was also capable of responding with rage. For example, when inadvertently hurt during handling of the stomach tube, she would push, kick, cry loudly and show other signs of vigorous resistance or evasion.

It was possible to induce depressive reactions experimentally by having a stranger enter the room and approach her. This reaction consisted of a cessation of most physical movements and a general flaccidity of muscles. She would turn her head away or face straight ahead. Her face sagged flabbily, the corners of the mouth went down, the inner parts of the eyebrows were elevated and brows were furrowed, producing an impression in an observer of deep melancholy. Usually she was silent but sometimes she would whimper. When the reaction was severe she would eventually close her eyes and fall asleep.

This depressive reaction was repeatedly induced, and recorded by observers behind one-way mirrors, on many occasions by the introduction of a stranger. If a person with a previously established positive relationship was present the depressive reaction was less severe but still occurred.

It is a plausible hypothesis that Monica developed some degree of normal responsiveness during her first five months but subsequently experienced continuing frustration of her needs for affection and nurturance— with the ultimate development of the depressive reaction, a reaction that by learning processes that are not entirely clear, came to be especially elicited by strangers. Perhaps the normal "fear-of-strangers" reaction that would ordinarily have developed within a month or two after her first depressive reaction played a role in facilitating a learned association between strangers and the depressive reaction.

There have been many anecdotal reports of grief reactions in animals following separation from a mate, child, parent, or human master. Nonhuman primates, especially, show a sequence of grief reactions remarkably similar to those seen in humans. Fortunately, in recent years there have been experimental studies with monkeys to supplement the anecdotal reports (Hinde, Spencer-Booth, & Bruce, 1966; Kaufman & Rosenblum, 1967; and Seay & Harlow, 1965). Kaufman and Rosenblum, for example, separated four infant monkeys from their mothers. Before separation the monkeys were reared in a group composed of the mother, the father, and another adult female. During separation, which lasted for four weeks, the infants remained with father and the other adult female. This procedure avoids confounding separation from mother with being put in a strange environment, a confounding that is present in most studies with human children (Bowlby, 1960; Freud & Burlingham, 1943; and Heinicke, 1956), except for Spitz's study (1946) in which the infants remained in the same environment during the mother's absence.

The immediate response to separation was vigorous protest involving loud screams, agitated pacing and searching, and a plaintive distress call referred to as cooing. This lasted for 24–36 hours, during which the infant did not sleep.

After 24–36 hours, there was a marked change in three of the four monkeys. These monkeys became inactive, stopped responding to or making social gestures, and ceased play behavior. They frequently sat hunched over, almost in a ball with head between their legs. The facial muscles sagged and they presented the classical facial configuration of human dejection. They occasionally emitted the plaintive cooing sound. Two of the monkeys developed autoerotic activity in the form of penis sucking—a reaction not seen in this monkey colony before except in one case of unplanned separation from the mother.

This depression-withdrawal phase lasted about five to six days, after which the monkeys gradually began to recover. The posture became more upright, exploration of the inanimate environment began, and a gradual increase in contacts with other monkeys occurred. For a while there were periods of depression that alternated with periods of exploration and play. By the end of the month of separation the infants had almost returned to normal. The recovery tendencies in these monkeys contrasts with the progressive deterioration and lack of recovery reported by Spitz for human infants. Whether this reflects a difference in species, in developmental level, or in conditions of separation (Spitz does not describe his procedures in sufficient detail) cannot be determined at this time.

Physiological Concomitants of Grief

There is little doubt that the initial protest phase is associated with general physiological arousal, probably including both sympathetic and parasympathetic autonomic reactions as well as arousal of the adrenocortical system. There is some controversy with respect to the nature of the physiological concomitants of the depression-withdrawal phase, that is, whether it is primarily a state of decreased physiological activity representing, perhaps, an attempt to conserve physiological resources, or whether it also involves some type of physiological arousal. Evidence rather strongly indicates that a marked decrease in gastrointestinal functioning accompanies grief. In the infant Monica, for example, hydrochloric acid secretion in the stomach was found to drop sharply during periods of depression. During active and joyful interaction with a familiar person hydrochloric secretion rate increased and was even higher during "rage" reactions. Other investigators have found similar inhibition in gastric secretion as well as salivation, stomach motility, and colonic functioning (Almy, 1951; Busfield & Wechsler, 1961; Kehoe & Ironside, 1963; and Wolff, 1953).

A decrease in these parasympathetic functions would be consistent with a general increase in sympathetic arousal. Findings, however, have been inconsistent with respect to an association between grief and sympathetic arousal (Averill, 1968).

There have been some consistent findings of increased adrenocortical functioning during grief. Friedman et al. (1963) found an increase in urinary products of adrenocortical hormones in the normal parents of children dying of leukemia during periods of acute stress, including the ultimate death of the child. Sachar et al. (1968) obtained daily measures of urinary indices of adrenocortical hormones in six women undergoing psychotherapy for depression (four were diagnosed as neurotic depression). During periods of confrontation with the precipitating loss, usually accompanied by an intensification of behavioral indications of grief, there were increases in indices of adrenocortical hormones. Both of these findings, however, might be interpreted as being more related to the protest phase of grief than to the depression-withdrawal stage. In the case of the women in psychotherapy the confrontations may be serving to arouse the person from the depression-withdrawal state and precipitate a protest reaction.

In conclusion the research so far suggests that the depression-withdrawal phase of grief is accompanied by less intense sympathetic arousal than is likely to be the case in fear, anger, or the protest phase of grief. Parasympathetic activity is decreased in the gastrointestinal tract and perhaps in other areas as well. The weeping response, however, is largely parasympathetic in nature, although weeping is not particularly common in the depressed-withdrawal stage. Adrenocortical functioning is undoubtedly increased during the protest phase and may continue to be elevated during depression-withdrawal.

One reason the results are not as clear as they might be is that the course of grief, whether normal or pathological, does not usually involve as sharp a delineation between protest and depression-withdrawal as we have implied. Although there may be periods of almost "pure" depression-withdrawal, it is likely that in most cases the period of protest is followed by a mixture of recurring protest reactions in which the person re-experiences the acute grief reaction and periods of depression-withdrawal. Measures of physiological response would probably vary as a function of the reaction which was prominent at the time. As we shall see in the next chapter, the picture is further complicated by various "defenses" that the person may employ to diminish this aversive experience. Taking these complications into account it may be reasonable to view the physiological aspects of grief in broad outline as one that begins with general autonomic and adrenocortical arousal and is followed by a depression-withdrawal period that reflects some degree of physiological exhaustion and an attempt at physiological conservation following the initial energy expenditure.

SHAME, GUILT, AND DISGUST

Is there a pattern of behavioral, physiological, and self-report responses that warrant the consideration of shame as a separate emotion from fear, anger, and grief? It seems probable, but the evidence is less clear than for the other types of emotional reaction. Behaviorally, shame is associated with hanging of the head and dropping the eyelid or averting the gaze. Physiologically, it is associated with blushing, a response in which the blood vessels of the skin (usually in the face and neck areas) are dilated to produce the characteristic reddening. Words such as shame, embarrassment, and humiliation are used to refer to the subjective experience accompanying this reaction. Most of us no doubt have a strong intuitive tendency to think of the subjective experience of embarrassment or humiliation as quite different from the subjective experiences that we label fear or grief. In the older child and adult the reaction of shame seems almost always to involve a situation in which some action or wish is exposed to the view of others. The action or wish usually involves a strong attraction, and the individual expects others to react with disapproval, perhaps in the form of ridicule or laughter. To be caught looking at someone with

sexual interest, or being greedy, selfish, or overly prideful are common circumstances that produce the shame reaction. There is thus an element of
secretive enjoyment that is discovered. If the discoverer is oneself, that is,
if one becomes aware of some action or wish in oneself that one strongly
disapproves, a shame reaction may occur. The latter reaction may be what
is commonly called *guilt;* I shall tentatively take the position that guilt is
the same reaction as shame, perhaps combined with some features of grief
or fear. The primary distinction between shame and guilt, then, is in terms
of stimulus conditions that elicit the reaction, that is, whether other people, as opposed to oneself, produce the response.

Disgust is not prominent in our classification scheme for emotional reactions. I consider it to consist basically of responses elicited by unsa-
vory smells and tastes, and to have close ties with the vomiting response.
In everyday usage the word disgust is used to cover a considerably wider
range of meanings than is intended here.

A distinctive and, for our purposes, important feature of fear, grief,
and shame is that all these reactions are unpleasant and the person will
tend to exert considerable effort to avoid or minimize the intensity, duration, and frequency of these reactions. I will in the future use the term
negative affect to refer generally to all emotions that are unpleasant or
aversive in this way.

In contrast to the negative affect of fear, grief, and shame, I postu-
late anger to be neither highly unpleasant nor pleasant. To the extent that
anger becomes associated with negative affects it can, of course, acquire
unpleasant features. It may be that one rarely experiences the emotion of
anger in isolation, for example, without thinking of aggressive actions that
could lead to consequences that would arouse negative affects such as fear,
grief, or shame. As we shall see in Chapter 6, strategies for avoiding negative affect play an important role in neurotic disorders. But I hypothesize
that anger tends to be avoided only when it is associated with an unpleasant outcome such as one of these unpleasant emotions.

Arbitrary interruptions (frustration) of ongoing behavioral sequences
are likely to instigate reactions of anger in animals and young children. It
is easy to see why the emotions of anger and grief occur together so frequently; both are likely to be elicited by physical or psychological depriva-
tions. Physiologically, anger tends to be accompanied by a strong sympathetic response, relatively high norepinephrine levels, and muscles tensed
for action. Physiological contrasts with the fear response were discussed
previously. The emotion of anger should be distinguished from overt goal-
directed behavior designed to hurt or destroy some object. I refer to sequences of the latter sort as *aggressive behavior.*

POSITIVE AFFECTS

Some emotional reactions are pleasant and enjoyable, and people expend effort and learn new ways to increase the intensity, duration, and frequency of such reactions. The emotional response of which smiling and laughter are a part would be an example. Excitement up to a point would be another example. In the latter case we speak of the pleasurable excitement associated with some anticipated event or the exhilarating excitement associated with a certain amount of danger that is successfully overcome, as in riding a roller coaster or parachute jumping. The ecstatic or mystical experience reported by some individuals, and some drug induced experiences, reflect variants of positive emotional reactions that we as yet know little about but are undoubtedly real. There are no sharp distinctions to be made between pleasurable emotions and the pleasures associated with satisfaction of the homeostatic drives such as eating, drinking, and sex.

CONCLUDING COMMENTS

Some background in the physiological bases of emotional reaction and some working definitions of emotional reactions such as fear, grief, shame, and anger have been provided. It is important to define and assess an emotional reaction in terms of all three available channels of information: behavioral, physiological, and self-report. Different emotions cannot be neatly packaged in precisely defined terms, since in reality human emotionality involves much variation in behavioral and physiological expression. The labels apply to loose classes of reaction that seem in our present state of knowledge to have important differences in function and expression. It is not likely that highly distinctive and separate neurophysiological systems will be found to be associated with these emotions. In later chapters we shall see how learning, the interplay of several emotions, and cognitive interpretations further complicate the phenomenon of emotional expression.

We are more likely to communicate accurately about emotional phenomena if we specify the actual procedures and measures from which we infer the presence of the emotion. Perhaps the greatest source of confusion in talking about emotions derives from the fact that we frequently use these labels in everyday speech. There is room for a great deal of individualized meaning in such usage; a person who says he is anxious to see a new movie is not referring to the same reaction as a person who says he is anxious about his impending execution. It is important, then, to remind ourselves continually that these terms as we have attempted to define them may not have exactly the same meaning as when we use them in ordinary conversation.

An implication of the greatest importance for the study of neurotic disorders is the extent to which the negative affects of fear, grief, and shame can be unpleasant. The subjective pain and agony that accompanies extreme reactions of these kinds can be almost unbearable, and this fact may explain much about the seeming irrationality of some neurotic behavior.

REFERENCES

Almy, T. P. Experimental studies on the irritable colon. *Amer. J. Med.,* 1951, **10,** 60–67.

Averill, J. R. Grief: Its nature and significance. *Psychol. Bull.,* 1968, **6,** 721–748.

Ax, A. F. The physiological differentiation between fear and anger in humans. *Psychosom. Med.,* 1953, **15,** 433–442.

Beam, J. C. Serial learning and conditioning under real life stress. *J. abnorm. soc. Psychol.,* 1955, **51,** 543–551.

Bitterman, M., & Holtzman, W. Conditioning and extinction of the galvanic skin response as a function of anxiety. *J. abnorm. soc. Psychol.,* 1952, **47,** 615–623.

Bowlby, J. Grief and mourning in infancy and early childhood. *Psychoanalytic study of the Child,* 1960, **15,** 9–52.

Busfield, B. L., & Wechsler, H. Studies of salivation in depression. *Arch. gen. Psychiat.,* 1961, **4,** 10–15.

Cannon, W. B. *Bodily changes in pain, hunger, fear and rage.* New York: Appleton, 1929.

Cohen, M. E., & White, P. D. Life situations, emotions and neurocirculatory asthenia (anxiety neurosis, neurasthenia, effort syndrome). *A Research nerv. & ment. Dis.,* 1950, 29, 832–869.

Davis, F. H., Malmo, R. B., & Shagass, C. Electromyographic reaction to strong auditory stimulation in psychiatric patients. *Canad. J. Psychol.,* 1954, **8,** 177–186.

Elmadjian, F., Hope, J. M., & Lamson, E. T. Excretion of epinephrine and norepinephrine in various emotional states. *J. Clin. Endocrinol.,* 1957, **17,** 608–620.

Engel, B. T. Stimulus-response and individual-response specificity. *Arch. gen. Psychiat.,* 1960, **2,** 305–313.

Engel, G. L., Reichsman, F., & Segal, H. L. A study of an infant with a gastric fistula. *Psychosom. Med.,* 1956, **5,** 374–398.

Frankenhaeuser, M., Jarpe, G., & Matell, G. Effects of intravenous infusions of adrenaline and noradrenaline on certain psychological and physiological functions. *Acta. Physiol. Scand.,* 1961, **51,** 175–186.

Franks, C. M. Conditioning and personality: A study of normal and neurotic subjects. *J. abnorm. soc. Psychol.,* 1956, **52,** 143–150.

Freud, A., & Burlingham, D. T. *War and children.* New York: Willard, 1943.

Friedman, S. B., Chodoff, P., Mason, J. W., & Hamburg, D. A. Behavioral observations on parents anticipating the death of a child. *Pediatrics,* 1963, **32**, 610–625.

Funkenstein, D. H., King, S. H., & Drolette, M. E. *Mastery of stress.* Cambridge: Harvard University Press, 1957.

Gellhorn, E. *Principles of autonomic-somatic integrations.* Minneapolis: University of Minnesota Press, 1967.

Harlow, H. F. The nature of love. *Amer. Psychol.,* 1958, **13**, 673–685.

Hebb, D. O. On the nature of fear. *Psychol. Rev.,* 1946, **53**, 259–276.

Heinicke, C. M. Some effects of separating two-year-old children from their parents: A comparative study. *Hum. Relat.,* 1956, **9**, 105–176.

Hinde, R. A., Spencer-Booth, Y., & Bruce, M. Effects of 6-day maternal deprivation on rhesus monkey infants. *Nature,* 1966, **210**, 1021–1023.

Jones, M., & Mellersh, V. Comparison of exercise response in anxiety states and normal controls. *Psychosom. Med.,* 1946, **8**, 180–187.

Kaufman, I. C., & Rosenblum, L. A. The reaction to separation in infant monkeys: Anaclitic depression and conservation-withdrawal. *Psychosom. Med.,* 1967, **29**, 648–675.

Kehoe, M., & Ironside, W. Studies on the experimental evocation of depressive responses using hypnosis: II. The influence of depressive responses upon secretion of gastric acid. *Psychosom. Med.,* 1967, **29**, 648–675.

Kelly, D. H. W. Measurement of anxiety by forearm blood flow. *Brit. J. Psychiat.,* 1966, **112**, 789–798.

Kelly, D. H. W., & Walter, C. J. S. The relationship between clinical diagnosis and anxiety, assessed by forearm blood flow and other measurements. *Brit. J. Psychiat.,* 1968, **114**, 611–626.

Lacey, J. T., Bateman, D. E., & Van Lehn, R. Autonomic response specificity. *Psychosom. Med.,* 1953, **15**, 8–21.

Lader, M. H. Palmar skin conductance measures in anxiety and phobic states. *J. psychosom. Res.,* 1967, **11**, 271–281.

Lader, M. H., & Wing, Lorna. Habituation of the psycho-galvanic reflex in patients with anxiety states and in normal subjects. *J. neurol., neurosurg., Psychiat.,* 1964, **27**, 210–218.

Lindeman, E. Symptomatology and management of acute grief. *Amer. J. Psychiat.,* 1944, **101**, 141–148.

Malmo, R. B. Studies of anxiety: Some clinical origins of the activation concept. In C. D. Spielberger (Ed.) *Anxiety and behavior.* New York: Academic Press, 1966.

Malmo, R. B., & Shagass, C. Studies of blood pressure in psychiatric patients under stress. *Psychosom. Med.,* 1952, **14**, 82–93.

Malmo, R. B., Shagass, C., & Davis, F. H. A method for the investigation of somatic response mechanisms in psychoneurosis. *Science,* 1950, **112**, 325–328.

Malmo, R. B., Shagass, C., & Heslam, R. M. Blood pressure response to repeated brief stress in psychoneurosis: A study of adaptation. *Canad. J. Psychol.,* 1951, **5**, 167–179.

Marris, P. *Widows and their families.* London: Routledge and Kegan Paul, 1958.

Persky, H., Korchin, S. J., Basowitz, H., Board, F. A., Sabshin, M., Hambrug, D. A., & Grinker, R. R. Effect of two psychological stresses on adrenocortical function. *A.M.A. Arch. Neurol. Psychiat.*, 1959, **81**, 103–110.

Pitts, F. N., & McClure, J. N. Lactate metabolism in anxiety neurosis. *New England J. Med.*, 1967, **277**, 1329–1336.

Richmond, J. B., & Lustman, S. L. Autonomic function in the neonate: implications for psychoanalytic theory. *Psychosom. Med.*, 1955, **17**, 269–275.

Rubin, L. S. Autonomic dysfunction in neurotic behavior. *Arch. gen. Psychiat.*, 1965, **12**, 572–585.

Sachar, E. J., Mackenzie, J. M., Binstock, W. A., & Mack, J. E. Corticosteroid responses to the psychotherapy of reactive depressions: II. Further clinical and physiological implications. *Psychosom. Med.*, 1968, **30**, 23–44.

Sackett, G. P. Monkeys reared in isolation with pictures as visual input: Evidence for an innate releasing mechanism. *Science*, 1966, **154**, 1468–1473.

Sainsbury, P. Muscle responses: Muscle tension and expressive movements. *J. psychosom. Res.*, 1964, **8**, 179–186.

Schachter, J. Pain, fear and anger in hypertensives and normotensives. *Psychosom. Med.*, 1957, **19**, 17–29.

Seay, B., & Harlow, H. F. Maternal separation in the rhesus monkey. *J. nerv. ment. Dis.*, 1965, **140**, 434–441.

Shagass, C., & Jones, A. L. A neurophysiological test for psychiatric diagnosis: Results in 750 Patients. *Amer. J. Psychiat.*, 1957, **114**, 1002–1009.

Silverman, A. J., & Cohen, S. I. Affect and vascular correlates to catecholamines. In L. J. West and M. Greenblatt (Eds.), *Explorations in the physiology of emotions*. Psychiatric Research Reports of the A.P.A., No. 12, January, 1960.

Spence, K. W. Anxiety (drive) level and performance in eyelid conditioning. *Psychol. Bull.*, 1964, **61**, 129–139.

Spitz, R. A. Hospitalism. *The Psychoanalytic Study of the Child*, 1945, **1**, 53–74.

Spitz, R. A. Anaclitic depression. *The Psychoanalytic Study of the Child*, 1946, **2**, 313–342.

Tomkins, E. H., Sturgis, C. C., & Wearn, J. T. Studies in epinephrine. II *A.M.A. Arch. Int. Med.*, 1919, **24**, 247–268.

Welsh, L., & Kubis, J. F. Conditioned PGR (psychogalvanic response) in states of pathological anxiety. *J. nerv. ment. Dis.*, 1947, **105**, 372–381.

Wolff, H. G. *Stress and disease*. Springfield, Ill.: Charles C. Thomas, 1953.

CHAPTER FOUR

HEREDITY

Almost all biological systems (anatomical, biochemical, neurological) are characterized by wide variations from individual to individual, and there is growing evidence that many of these individual differences are influenced by hereditary (genetic) factors (e.g., Williams, 1956). Some of these genetically influenced characteristics may be especially relevant to the development of neurotic disorder. Autonomic nervous system reactivity and sociability are two likely candidates for this role. If a person inherited a tendency toward unusually strong autonomic reactivity, perhaps associated with greater ease of autonomic conditioning, it is easy to see how he might be more susceptible to the development of anxiety, phobic, and perhaps obsessive-compulsive reactions.

MEASURING HEREDITARY INFLUENCE

Biological inheritance is transmitted by genes and the totality of these genes for a given individual is referred to as the genotype. We cannot, by present methods, directly measure genotypes. The observable characteristics of an individual, whether physical or behavioral, are referred to as the phenotype. The phenotype is *not inherited*, but is the result of a given genotype interacting with given environmental circumstances. Thus observable characteristics from birth on represent an interaction between genotype and environment that cannot be readily unraveled, and it does not ordinarily make sense to say that something is caused by heredity or caused by environment. On the other hand, it is clearly the case that heredity plays a more influential role in producing individual differences in certain phenotypic characteristics than in others: for example, eye color as opposed to the particular language spoken.

The most useful procedure for assessing hereditary influence in humans is to compare degree of similarity in identical and same-sex fraternal twin pairs. Identical twins are born with identical genotypes and fraternal twins are born with no greater similarity in genotype than ordinary siblings. Since in both cases the twins grow up in very similar environments (same parents, siblings, and neighborhood), differences in degree of similarity between identical and fraternal twins are largely due to the greater hereditary similarity in the identical twins. The only problem with this interpretation is that identical twins because of their greater physical likeness may actually experience greater similarity in environmental response than fraternal twins. For example, other people might not be able to tell them apart with much certainty and thus respond similarly to both.

ANIMAL RESEARCH

The possibility that dispositions to "nervousness" and sociability might be inherited would not be surprising to anyone familiar with animal breeding. Dogs, for example, have been bred to accentuate all kinds of personality traits. In a controlled breeding experiment using purebred pointers Murphree and Dykman (1965) were able to produce strains of fearful or friendly dogs within a couple of generations. Some dogs were separated from their mother at birth so that differences in these cases could not be explained in terms of learning from the mother. In standardized tests fearful dogs showed less exploratory activity in a free situation, less approach to humans, and more posturing and freezing in response to a noise. These "fear" reactions did not occur until the dogs were 40–60 days of age, suggesting the role of maturational processes.

AUTONOMIC REACTIVITY

Jost and Sontag (1944) found identical twins to be more alike on autonomic measures than sibling pairs. Vandenberg, Clark, and Samuels (1965) found identical twins to be more alike on heart rate response than fraternal twins. And Block (1967) found very high similarity in a group of identical twins on measures of heart rate and palmar skin resistance. He did not, however, provide comparisons with a group of fraternal twins.

In perhaps the best autonomic study reported to date Lader and Wing (1966) compared 11 pairs of identical twins with 11 pairs of same sex fraternal twins (all 17 to 26 years old) on measures obtained during the presentation of a series of 20 tones. The procedure was described in Chapter 3, p. 30. Results from studies of this kind are frequently presented in the form of correlations, a statistic that ranges from -1.0 to $+1.0$ and indicates degree of relationship between two measures. In this case a positive correlation means that if one twin of a pair has a high score on a given measure, then the other twin is also likely to have a high score, and likewise if one twin has a low score, the other twin is likely to have a low score. The magnitude of the correlation indicates the degree of similarity among the twin pairs. Skin conductance change from beginning to end of the session showed essentially the same correlation for the two twin groups, .52 and .51. A measure of the tendency for galvanic skin responses (GSR's) to decrease (habituate) with the successive presentation of tones yielded a correlation of .75 for identical twins and .13 for fraternal twins. A measure of frequency of nonspecific or spontaneous GSR's obtained near the end of the session correlated .68 for identical twins and $-.02$ for fraternal twins. Heart rate near the end of the session correlated .78 for identical twins and $-.38$ (probably a chance difference from zero) for the fraternal twins. Similar measures were found to discriminate anxiety reaction patients from normal controls in studies reported in Chapter 3 (Lader & Wing, 1964; Lader, 1967).

The above studies rather strongly indicate a hereditary component in autonomic reactivity. More research is needed to give a clearer picture of the magnitudes of the hereditary factor. Specifically, it would be desirable to have larger samples of younger children (so that differences in environmental experiences can be minimized) and to use a greater range of autonomic and adrenocortical measures under varying conditions of stimulation and stress.

SOCIABILITY

Sociability and extraversion-introversion are used interchangeably in the following discussion to refer to the dimension represented at one end by individuals who are shy and socially fearful, especially with respect to strangers or new social situations, and at the other end to individuals who are outgoing, expansive, and at ease in new as well as established social situations. A hereditary component in sociability has been suggested by several studies comparing identical and fraternal twins. Gottesman (1962,

1966) reported two such studies. In the first study, 34 pairs of identical and same-sex fraternal adolescent twins were compared on six scales from a self-report questionnaire, the Minnesota Multiphasic Personality Inventory (MMPI). One of these scales was the Social Introversion scale composed of the following kinds of items: I am a good mixer; I like to go to parties and other affairs where there is lots of loud fun. The correlation between identical twin pairs on this scale was .55 and between fraternal twins, .08. Gottesman found similar results in the second study.

Scarr (1965) reported a study using younger twins, all girls, between the ages of six and ten. Twenty-four pairs of identical twins were compared with 28 pairs of fraternal twins on ratings of social apprehension based on home observations. The correlation between pairs of identical twins was .88, between fraternal twins, .28.

Freedman and Keller (1963) obtained behavior ratings in the homes, every month for their first year, on 9 identical and 12 fraternal twins. Measures based on the 21-item Bayley Infant Behavior Profile, which included several sociability and fearfulness items, showed greater average similarity for the identical than for the fraternal twins. These ratings were made from separate movies of each twin. One group of judges made the ratings for one twin and another group of judges made the ratings for the co-twin, thus avoiding "halo" effects from knowing which twins belonged together. It is unlikely that at this early age similarity between twins has been much influenced by mutual imitation of each other. The only drawback to this study is that results for the individual 21 items were not presented so one cannot be sure that the results apply specifically to sociability as opposed to other items involving such characteristics as activity level and attention span.

Shields (1962) compared 42 identical twins separated early in life and reared apart with 43 identical twins reared together and with 25 fraternal twins reared together on a self-report Extraversion-Introversion scale. The correlation between identical twins reared apart was .61, identical twins reared together, .42, and fraternal twins reared together, −.17. These results not only indicate a significant heredity factor but also suggest that any greater environmental similarity experienced by the identical twins reared together did not increase their similarity on extraversion-introversion since the correlation was actually lower for the twins reared together than for those reared apart. An interesting observation reported in this study is that the close relationship between the twins may in itself produce a *lack* of similarity on any traits involving social dominance. In a close twin relationship if one twin becomes somewhat dominant the other is likely to reciprocate by being somewhat submissive. This, at least, is probably a more likely outcome than a continuing struggle for dominance. The result is that twins reared together would be less alike on social dominance (very much involved in most measures of extraversion-introversion) than those reared apart where inherited influences on social dominance would not be affected by dynamics of the twin relationship.

Kagan and Moss (1962) found consistent individual differences in sociability and social dominance from early childhood to adolescence. Relatively high consistency over time would be expected in a trait with some hereditary component.

NEUROTIC DISORDER

Shields (1954) obtained samples from the general population of 36 identical and 26 same-sex fraternal twins, ages 12 to 15 years. On the basis of parent interviews, neurotic characteristics present in each twin were counted and each twin was then placed in one of four categories according to degree of severity of the symptom. In category one, moderately severe, were included all twins who had been taken to a child guidance clinic on account of nervous symptoms, or who had enuresis that had continued beyond the age of eight, or who had symptoms of marked shyness, night terrors, phobias, and delinquency. This range of symptoms involves a rather broad definition of neurosis, and delinquency is especially questionable as a neurotic symptom. At the other end, category four involved a complete absence of neurotic characteristics.

Twenty-five percent of the identical and 8 percent of the fraternal twins were rated as being in the same category, indicating greater similarity for identical twins. Shields then made more refined ratings of degree of similarity in terms of kind of symptom, not just degrees of severity. Thirty-six percent of the identical and zero percent of the fraternal twins were "completely concordant", 17 percent of the identical and 69 percent of the fraternal twins were discordant, and the remaining twins represented various degrees of partial concordance. These findings certainly suggest greater similarity on neurotic characteristics in identical twins. Unfortunately, the author did not assess the reliability (agreement by independent raters) of his ratings, and there is no indication that the ratings were made without knowledge of the identical or fraternal status of the twins or the nature of the symptoms present in the co-twin. Shields does give some interesting case examples of discordant identical twins where birth difficulty or organic disease in one twin seems to have provided a basis for differential development, and other cases where different parental response seems to have been the primary factor.

Over 50 percent of these twins fell in categories 1 or 2 (moderate or mild severity). This may seem like a high incidence of disorder for the general population but probably reflects the relative mildness of the symptoms being counted and also the likelihood that a high proportion of children do experience some type of disturbance in the process of growing up, which is usually overcome and does not lead to serious handicap in adult life. Thomas et al. (1968) report a similar incidence of disturbance in younger children from "normal" families.

Anxiety Reaction

Slater and Shields (1969) report concordance percentages on 17 identical and 28 same-sex fraternal twins, average age of 40 years, where one of the twins, called the *proband,* had been diagnosed as anxiety reaction. Forty-one percent of the identical co-twins and 4 percent of the fraternal co-twins had received a diagnosis of anxiety reaction. If cases were included whose primary diagnosis was not anxiety reaction but who nevertheless had marked anxiety traits, then the percentage concordance figures rose to 65 percent and 13 percent, respectively. These results in conjunction with the evidence presented previously for a hereditary influence on autonomic reactivity and sociability strongly suggest a hereditary component in anxiety reactions. It is a plausible hypothesis that individuals with an inherited tendency to be autonomically reactive and socially apprehensive represent a higher than average risk group for the later development of anxiety reactions. Whether they do so depends on environmental experiences.

Hysteria

Slater (1961) found no difference in concordance rates for 12 identical and 12 fraternal twin pairs where one twin had received a diagnosis of hysteria. No co-twins of either type had received a clear cut diagnosis of hysteria. Five identical and 4 fraternal co-twins might be considered as concordant for a neurotic disorder of some kind, but not specifically for hysteria. The lack of a meaningful difference in concordance between identical and fraternal pairs argues against a hereditary component in hysteria. Gottesman (1962) also failed to find differences in degree of similarity between identical and fraternal high school age twins on the Hysteria Scale of the MMPI. There is some question, however, as to whether individual differences in the general population on the MMPI Hysteria Scale are directly related to neurotic symptoms of conversion (paralysis, blindness, deafness, etc.) and dissociation. Conversion and dissociative reactions tend to have an "all or none" character as opposed to the more continuous variations found for anxiety. Individuals do not tend to have "small" paralyses or "small" amnesic episodes that become accentuated to form the final neurotic symptom in the same way that an anxiety-prone person may develop more acute anxiety attacks.

Depression

The role of hereditary factors in depression is not clear. This lack of clarity stems in part from the continuing uncertainty as to whether the difference between neurotic and psychotic depressions represents only differences in severity along a common dimension or different disorders with distinctive symptom patterns and causes. There is some evidence that the psychotic (sometimes referred to as endogenous) depressions have hereditary components but that neurotic or reactive depressions do not (Shields & Slater, 1961; Slater & Shields, 1969). In the latter study, 8 identical and 16 same-sex fraternal twins were compared where the probands had all been diagnosed as having neurotic depressions. None of the co-twins of either type, identical or fraternal, had received a similar diagnosis.

ORGANIC DISEASE AND HYSTERIA

Consideration of hereditary factors in hysteria is further complicated by the problem of distinguishing between symptoms produced by organic disease and those produced by genetic or learning factors. Slater and Glithero (1965) conducted a nine-year follow-up study of patients initially diagnosed with hysteria and found that 60% had either died from or developed signs of physical disease during this period. A high proportion of the diseases involved the central nervous system. Kiersch (1962) intensively studied 98 cases of amnesia in military personnel at a general army hospital. Forty-one were found to be feigning the loss of memory, that is, malingering; 20 were caused by psychological factors; 24 were caused by organic brain disease or acute alcoholism; and 13 were considered to be a mixture of at least two of the above. The approximately 25% found to be suffering from a definite organic disorder is less than that reported by Slater and Glithero but is still substantial. It is also quite possible that if Kiersch were able to reexamine these patients nine years later, as Slater and Glithero did, the proportion of organic brain disorders would increase.

Whitlock (1967) compared the incidence of organic brain disorder in 56 patients who were diagnosed as hysterical with 56 patients who were diagnosed as depressive and/or as having anxiety reactions. In 62.5% of the hysteria patients there was evidence indicative of organic brain disorder, as compared with 5.3% of the depression and/or anxiety patients. The most common indication of possible brain disorder in the hysteria patients was a head injury with concussion occurring within six months prior to the onset of this conversion or dissociative symptom. Other kinds of organic brain disorders present included cerebro-vascular accident (stroke), epilepsy, encephalitis, and brain tumor. This study is of particular interest because it also shows the relatively low proportion of organic brain disorders in neurotic symptoms other than hysteria.

Some conversion symptoms such as "glove" anesthesias or paralyses without other neurological signs are likely to be hysterical in nature because they represent conditions that are almost impossible to achieve by any known neurological disorder. Unfortunately, it is frequently difficult to rule out organic causation in many other hysterical symptoms by current neurological procedures. It may be several years before the organic disease process will become detectable neurologically as was found in the Slater and Glithero (1965) study. It is also likely that in some cases the symptom results from a combination of psychological and brain disorder factors. For example, head injury with concussion is very likely to involve psychological trauma as well as organic brain trauma. It is not possible to obtain a clear picture of the role of heredity by twin studies unless most of the cases with organic brain disease have been eliminated from the twin samples. For example, Slater (1961) discovered that several of the twins used in his study probably had brain disease.

CONCLUSIONS

We conclude, then, that there is considerable evidence that autonomic reactivity and sociability are influenced by hereditary factors. Likewise there is evidence from twin studies that hereditary factors contribute to the development of anxiety reactions. These results do not tell us just how individual differences in autonomic reactivity and sociability might eventuate in the full-blown anxiety reaction. Evidence at this time does not support a conclusion that heredity plays a role in neurotic depression or hysteria.

THE INTERACTION OF HEREDITY AND SOCIAL LEARNING

If hereditary predispositions do exist, they are undoubtedly influenced by environmental learning experiences starting at birth. Thomas, Chess, and Birch (1968) report a study that illustrates the interaction between traits thought to be influenced by heredity and social learning experiences. In this research the development of 136 children was followed from birth to ages 6–12 in 85 families. The families were of middle and upper middle class background and lived in New York City or a surrounding suburb. The investigators were especially interested in assessing individual differences in temperament that were present in the first year or so of life and presumed to be largely inherited, and in seeing how these temperamental characteristics affected later personality development. Measures of child behavior and temperament were obtained by parent interviews at 3-month intervals during the first 18 months of life, at 6-month intervals until 5 years, and at yearly intervals thereafter. The interviews emphasized factual descriptions of recent or current behavior. The validity of the interview data was checked by home observations of child behavior on a subsample of families. Other sources of data included school observations, teacher interviews and standardized psychological tests.

In the course of the study, 42 of the children developed mildly to moderately severe behavior disorders and were seen more intensively by the staff. Thus, the study provides an opportunity to see what kind of temperamental characteristics were present in these children *before* the onset of the behavior disturbances—an unusual circumstance in psychopathology research.

When the children were still less than two years of age the investigators had identified a subgroup of 14 children that they labeled "difficult children." Prominent temperamental characteristics of these children were as follows: 1) biological irregularity, especially with respect to sleep, feeding, and elimination cycles; 2) withdrawal and associated expressions of distress to new stimuli, for example, to the first bath, to new foods, new people or new places; 3) slow adaptability to change, taking many exposures to new situations before overcoming the initial negative reaction, and 4) a predominance of negative mood, involving a greater readiness to fuss and cry with high intensity. Seventy percent (10 cases) of these difficult children subsequently developed behavior disorders. The overall incidence of behavior disorders in the total sample was about 31 percent. The finding thus suggests that these early temperamental traits contributed to the subsequent development of behavior disorder.

The parents of the difficult children did not differ from the parent group as a whole in their approach to child care during the early years as measured by interviews. However, in a number of cases, as the difficult child grew older, disturbances in parent-child interaction emerged that appeared to be reactive to the special characteristics of these children. Many of these college-educated mothers reacted to the troublesome features of the child with self-blame; for example, by interpreting their child's difficult behavior in terms of psychodynamic theories in which the mother's unconscious attitude of rejection must be producing the problem. Other parents interpreted the child's crying and irregularity as being intentionally defiant and reacted punitively. The development of child disturbance is traced in a number of families in a way that highlights the interaction between child predisposition and parent reaction.

The authors describe two difficult children that were very similar in temperamental make-up in the first few years of life. The two sets of parents, however, responded differently to the children and by age five and a half years one, a girl, had developed a marked behavioral disturbance including explosive anger, negativism, fear of the dark, encopresis (defecating in clothes), thumb sucking, insatiable demands for toys and sweets, poor peer relationships, and protective lying. The other child, a boy, developed no symptoms of behavior disorder. The father of the girl disciplined her in a punitive way and spent little or no recreational time with her. The mother was more understanding and more permissive but quite inconsistent. Adaptation to nursery school in the fourth year was a problem for both children, and the parents of the girl, especially the father, reacted angrily to her difficulties in adjusting to nursery school. The parents of the boy, on the other hand, were patient and tolerant of his slowness to adapt to new situations such as nursery school.

The findings of Thomas et al. would suggest that genetically influenced characteristics such as temperament traits or autonomic reactivity may or may not lead to neurotic disorder. That eventuality is largely dependent upon social learning experiences.

REFERENCES

Block, J. D. Monozygotic twin similarity in multiple psychophysiologic parameters and measures. In J. Wortis (Ed.), *Recent advances in biological psychiatry, Vol. 9*. New York: Plenum Press, 1967.

Freedman, D. G., & Keller, A. Inheritance of behavior in infants. Science, 1963, **140**, 196–198.

Gottesman, I. Differential inheritance of the psychoneuroses. *Eugen. Quart.*, 1962, **9**, 223–227.

Gottesman, I. Genetic variance in adaptive personality traits. *J. child psychol. & Psychiat.*, 1966, **7**, 199–208.

Jost, H., & Sontag, L. W. The genetic factor in autonomic nervous system function. *Psychosom. Med.*, 1944, **6**, 308–310.

Kagan, J., & Moss, H. A. *Birth to maturity: A study in psychological development.* New York: Wiley, 1962.

Kiersch, T. A. Amnesia: A clinical study of ninety-eight cases. *Amer. J. Psychiat.*, 1962, **119**, 57–60.

Lader, M. H. Palmer skin conductance measures in anxiety and phobic states. *J. psychosom. Res.*, 1967, **11**, 271–281.

Lader, M. H., & Wing, L. Habituation of the psycho-galvanic reflex in patients with anxiety states and in normal subjects. *J. neurol., neurosurg., Psychiat.*, 1964, **27**, 210–218.

Lader, M. H., & Wing, L. Physiological measures, sedative drugs, and morbid anxiety. *Maudsley Monographs No. 14*. London: Oxford Univ. Press, 1966.

Murphree, O. D., & Dykman, R. A. Litter patterns in the offspring of nervous and stable dogs. I: Behavioral tests. *J. nerv. ment. Dis.*, 1965, **141**, 321–332.

Scarr, S. The inheritance of sociability. Paper presented at American Psychological Association meeting in Chicago, September 5, 1965.

Shields, J. Personality differences and neurotic traits in normal twin school children. *Eugen. Rev.*, 1954, **45**, 213–245.

Shields, J. *Monozygotic twins, brought up apart and brought up together*. London: Oxford Univ. Press, 1962.

Shields, J., & Slater, E. Heredity and psychological abnormality. In H. J. Eysenck (Ed.), *Handbook of abnormal psychology*. New York: Basic Books, 1961.

Slater, E. The thirty-fifth Maudsley lecture: 'Hysteria 311'. *J. ment. Sci.*, 1961, **107**, 359–381.

Slater, E., & Glithero, E. A follow-up of patients diagnosed as suffering from hysteria. *J. psychosom. Res.*, 1965, **9**, 9–13.

Slater, E., & Shields, J. Genetical aspects of anxiety. In M. H. Lader (Ed.), *Studies of anxiety*. Ashford, Kent, England: Headley Bros., 1969.

Thomas, A., Chess, S., & Birch, H. G., *Temperament and behavior disorders in children*. New York: New York Univ. Press, 1968.

Vandenberg, S. G., Clark, P. J., & Samuels, I. Psychophysiological reactions of twins: Heritability factors in galvanic skin resistance, heartbeat, and breathing rates. *Eugen. Quart.*, 1965, **12**, 7–10.

Whitlock, F. A. The aetiology of hysteria. *Acta Psychiatrica Scandinavica* 1967, **43**, 144–162.

Williams, R. J. *Biochemical individuality*. New York: Wiley, 1956.

CHAPTER FIVE

LEARNING AND NEUROTIC DISORDER: BASIC CONCEPTS

It is not possible to consider the nature and development of neurotic disorders without reference to learning processes, especially learning processes involving emotional expression and social interaction. You are encouraged to review introductory sources if you are unsure of the meaning of any terminology being used.

There is considerable danger in taking a few terms and concepts from laboratory-based experiments on restricted aspects of the learning process and using them to interpret a complicated phenomenon such as neurotic disorder. Without the empirical research on the phenomenon itself this comes perilously close to an exercise in explaining by naming. It is especially seductive because we use terms that appear to have scientific respectability, such as conditioned stimuli, discriminative stimuli, and reinforcement—rather than terms like demon possession, Jungian archetypes, Freudian unconscious. The advantage of the research-based terminology is not that the complex phenomena of neurosis can with any certainty be completely explained in these terms, but that these terms are much more likely to suggest strategies of empirical research that will further our understanding of these disorders. And, perhaps most important, this objectively oriented terminology can suggest experiments that may *disprove* certain hypotheses, and thus require revision of the theory. The most damaging thing that can be said about certain aspects of the older theories of neurosis, such as those of Freud and Jung, is that they were not stated in language that made them susceptible to experimental disproof and consequent revision.

CLASSICAL CONDITIONING

Some familiarity with terminology and procedures associated with the classical conditioning paradigm is assumed; for example, conditioned stimulus (CS), unconditioned stimulus (UCS), unconditioned response (UCR), and conditioned response (CR). The classical conditioning model is most appropriately applied to the study of simple reflexes such as pupil constriction, saliva flow, and eyelid blinks. Since many of the autonomic responses associated with emotional reactions, such as the galvanic skin response and heart rate, seem to be susceptible to this kind of learning, the process is of some importance for neurotic disorder.

Experimenters are reluctant to use unduly stressful UCS with humans, and have usually employed mildly painful electric shock, so that conditioning effects tend to be rather weak and not to persist. There are, however, many studies in which autonomic responses in humans are shown to occur in situations, or in anticipation of situations, when it is reasonable to assume that conditioning to previously noneliciting stimuli has occurred in the past. Heart rate acceleration, for example, has been shown to occur during anticipation of oral examinations (Hickam, Cargill, & Golden, 1948), during verbal criticism (Malmo, Boag, & Smith, 1957), and in a situation in which the subject was led to believe that he might receive a dangerous electric shock (Ax, 1953). Shannon, Szmyd, and Prigmore (1962) found that measures of adrenocortical response increased during anticipation of dental procedures such as impaction surgery.

The responses associated with fear seem to be highly learnable on the basis of simple contiguity with previously noneliciting stimuli. When a sufficiently intense fear reaction has occurred, only a few, in some cases only one, pairing of the CS with the fear reaction is enough to produce a strong fear response when the individual encounters the CS in the future.

In an unusual study with human subjects Campbell, Sanderson, and Laverty (1964) used drug-induced respiratory paralysis as the UCS and a 600-cps tone as a CS. After habituation to the tone had occurred, six subjects, the experimental group, were given the respiratory-paralysis-inducing-drug paired with simultaneous presentation of the tone. Three subjects in one control group were given the UCS without tone, and three subjects in a second control group were given the tone without the UCS. The duration of the respiratory paralysis ranged from 90 to 130 seconds, and was described subsequently by the subjects as horrific. The respiratory paraly-

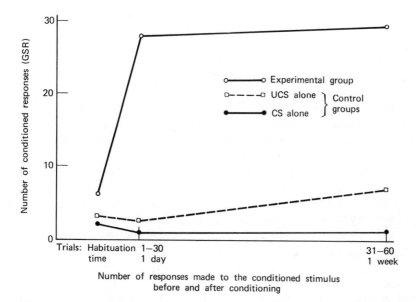

Number of responses made to the conditioned stimulus
before and after conditioning

FIGURE 6. Mean number of UCR and CR for experimental and control subjects during the habituation period and 60 extinction trials (Campbell, Sanderson, & Laverty, 1964).

sis was accompanied by general paralysis so that the totally conscious subjects experienced the frightening situation of not being able to breathe and at the same time being completely helpless physically. Many subsequently expressed the fear that they were going to die. Following paralysis subjects were allowed to settle down for about five minutes and then were given 30 five second presentations of the tone at varying intervals. No further induced paralyses were given. One week later all subjects were given 30 more trials with the tone, without the UCS.

The number of conditioned responses for the three groups during habituation, the 30 trials immediately following paralysis, and the 30 trials a week later are shown in Figure 6. It is clear that the one pairing of tone with paralysis produced a strong and persisting GSR to the tone. The subjects in the experimental group were given yet another series of 40 tones three weeks after the first session and still showed the same high rate of responding. Similar results were obtained for a measure of nonspecific GSR's, those that occurred "spontaneously" without any obvious association to the CS or other external stimuli. There was also a tendency for the latency of the GSR, that is, the time interval between onset of CS and the beginning of the GSR, to become shorter in the succeeding sessions for the experimental group. Heart rate responses presented more measurement difficulties but in general were similar to the GSR data.

This study shows the effectiveness of only one pairing of a CS and a strong fear response in producing a learned association. It is noteworthy that the authors found no evidence for extinction of the response to the nonreinforced CS over a three-week period and 100 presentations of the tone.

The long-lasting effects of one experience with naturally occurring traumatic events have been described by Kardiner (1943), with respect to soldiers in dangerous combat situations, and Leopold and Dillon (1963), with respect to a disastrous marine explosion that occurred on March 7, 1957. A gasoline tanker, the *Mission San Francisco,* collided with *Elna II,* a freighter, in the Delaware River. An intense explosion occurred and 10 men were killed. Many of the survivors of this traumatic experience were given a psychiatric examination at the time and again about four years later. Most of the survivors reported symptoms of one kind or another: emotional disturbances involving nervousness, tension, and general upset; sleep disturbances; and gastrointestinal disturbances. In general there was a tendency for the number of disturbances to *increase* over the four-year period. Many were unable to return to sea on a regular basis and most of those who did indicated that they were tense and fearful aboard ship but that going to sea was a matter of occupational necessity. A control group that had not had the traumatic experience would have been desirable in this study as a check on the general tendency for symptomology to increase with time or age, but it is clear that the trauma survivors did not show much "spontaneous" decrease in their fear-related symptoms over this four-year period.

There may be some slight support for an *incubation effect,* that is, a tendency for fear to increase with the passage of time without intervening contact with the feared situation, in the Campbell et al., and Leopold & Dillon studies. Experimental demonstration of incubation effects is still equivocal, although much folklore seems based on an assumption of this kind. One is told, for example, to get back immediately on a horse after being thrown off; otherwise the fear will grow and one will never be able to ride again.

Watson and Rayner (1920) conducted a study with a one-year-old infant that has long been cited in textbooks as a demonstration of the conditionability of fear in humans. Albert had been living in a hospital environment with a wet-nurse for a mother almost from birth. He was described as an unusually healthy and unemotional child. Before conditioning he had been shown an array of objects, most of which involved some furriness, such as a white rat, a rabbit, a dog, and cotton wool. He showed no signs of fear in their presence.

As a fear-inducing UCS the investigators used an unexpected noise produced by striking a steel bar sharply close behind the infant. In the first session the bar was struck on two occasions when Albert reached out to touch a white rat. A week later, five more paired presentations of rat and noise were given. On the eighth trial the rat alone was presented and Albert immediately began to cry and crawled away rapidly. Five days later he was tested for generalization of the fear response. He played as usual with wooden blocks, showing no sign of fear. When the rabbit was put in front of him he responded at once, leaning as far away from the animal as possible, whimpering, and finally bursting into tears. Similar, but less strong, reactions were obtained to the dog, cotton wool, and other furry objects. Watson and Rayner had planned to "recondition" Albert by providing pleasant feeding experiences in the presence of the rat, but circumstances led to his unavoidable removal from the hospital at this time.[1]

In summary, the three studies described above support the conclusions that an intense fear experience is readily conditionable to stimuli that happen to be present at the time, and that such conditioned fear tends to persist over long periods of time.

INSTRUMENTAL LEARNING

In instrumental or operant learning the organism learns to make a response that is instrumental in effecting a change in the environment, usually in the form of providing a reinforcement for the organism.

Reinforcement and discriminative stimuli. Reinforcement is defined empirically as an event that happens after the instrumental response that tends to increase the probability of occurrence of the response when the same discriminative stimuli are present on future occasions. A stimulus that precedes a number of pairings of an instrumental response with subsequent reinforcement can come to serve as a discriminative stimulus. Such a discriminative stimulus can be thought of as a signal that tells the organism that making a certain response will yield a certain reinforcement. The only way to determine whether a given stimulus is actually serving as a discriminative stimulus is to see if its presence *does* increase the probability of the response. A child observes a sibling receive a cookie (the discriminative stimulus); the child yells, "I want one too" (the instrumental response); and the child is given a cookie (the reinforcement). On subsequent occasions this particular discriminative stimulus is more likely to

---

[1] I have serious reservations about the use of respiratory paralysis with adult human subjects and the experimental arousal of strong fear in infants. In any experimentation with human subjects it is essential to provide complete information about any possible harmful experiences and obtain the subject's consent. Young children and infants should not be used as subjects if harmful effects are likely to occur.

elicit this particular instrumental response.

We also have no sure way of knowing ahead of time whether a given event will be reinforcing, with the possible exception of certain techniques of direct stimulation in the limbic systems of the brain (Olds, 1969). In general, providing the appropriate gratification for organisms deprived of water, food, sex, and other biological needs is reinforcing. The reinforcement in these cases is essentially unlearned or innate, and we refer to them as primary reinforcers. Certain stimuli, by virtue of their close association with primary reinforcement, especially when they serve as discriminative stimuli predicting the future occurrence of primary reinforcement, can come to serve as reinforcers themselves. We speak of these as secondary or learned reinforcers. The presence of mother, her smile, and, later, verbal indications of her praise or approval usually become learned reinforcers. In the adult world money, signs of social approval, or status recognition are all powerful learned reinforcers. Research indicates, however, that learned reinforcers will ultimately lose their reinforcing power if all association with primary reinforcers is discontinued for a long enough period.

Reinforcement may occur not only with attainment of some "desired" object, but also can occur as the result of the removal or escape from some aversive or unpleasant stimulation. Thus the removal of or escape from a painful stimulus, such as a loud noise or extreme heat, tends to be reinforcing for the response that precedes it. The terms *punishment* and *aversive consequence* are used interchangeably in future discussions.

AVOIDANCE LEARNING

The concept of avoidance learning is important in understanding neurotic disorders, especially when such learning allows a person to avoid situations that elicit strong fear, grief, or shame reactions. In these circumstances it is likely that the person has experienced in his past history some combination of classical conditioning and instrumental avoidance learning. Fear, for example, may first have become conditioned to certain stimuli. Subsequently the person learns to escape from these fear-eliciting stimuli, and this escape response is reinforced by removal or reduction of the aversive fear experience. Note that we are assuming a hypothetical fear response that is aversive. There is no external application of an aversive stimulus such as painful electric shock, loud noise, intense cold, etc. If certain other stimuli serve as discriminative stimuli that permit one to predict ahead of time the occurrence of the fear-eliciting stimuli, then one may learn to avoid these stimuli and the associated fear response altogether.

Avoidance learning in which strong aversive stimuli are used can result in responses that are unusually resistant to extinction. Solomon and his associates have performed a series of experiments with dogs using the avoidance learning paradigm. Solomon, Kamin, and Wynne (1953) employed a shuttle box with two compartments separated by a gate. The CS consisted of turning a light off over the compartment in which the dog happened to be. The light stayed off until the dog jumped over the gate into the lighted compartment. The US consisted of an intense electric shock applied through the grid floor, and was started ten seconds after onset of the CS. The dogs readily learned to jump over the gate to avoid shock, and were then placed on extinction for 200 trials; that is, no shock was given even if the dog delayed longer than 10 seconds in jumping. There was no tendency for the response to extinguish; in fact the average latency of response decreased over 200 trials. In a previous pilot experiment the authors had found that a dog continued for 490 extinction trials with no sign of extinction.

The strength of the avoidance response was further demonstrated in a second experiment in the Solomon, Kamin, and Wynne study. Nine dogs were trained in essentially the same procedure as previously described. After the 200 extinction trials a glass barrier that prevented jumping was interposed between compartments on four of the 10 trials for 10 straight days. The dogs were thus forced to remain in the compartment and have the opportunity to learn that shock was no longer forthcoming. Seven of the nine dogs failed to extinguish in the 100 trials given under this condition. In a third experiment 13 dogs were given similar initial training, and then the dogs were shocked for three seconds for jumping into the other compartment, the previously learned avoidance response. Ten of the 13 dogs failed to extinguish in 100 shock-extinction trials of this kind. In fact, the dogs tended to jump faster after shock-extinction was introduced than before. In a paradoxical way shock or punishment for the response seems to have strengthened it!

In a fourth experiment a combination of glass barrier and shock-extinction was used with dogs that had not extinguished under the conditions in the previous experiments. With this combined procedure the dogs finally stopped making the avoidance response after about seven days.

The extreme persistence of responses that have been learned to avoid strong aversive stimulation has been demonstrated in other experiments, for example, in rats by Miller (1951). Mowrer (1950) suggested that avoidance learning was based on two processes: classical conditioning of an aversive emotional response such as fear; and an instrumental response that removes the animal from the stimuli that elicit the aversive emotional response. Solomon and Wynne (1954) suggest that Mowrer's account does not completely explain the extreme persistence of avoidance learning based on strongly aversive stimuli. They propose that the classically conditioned fear response is *partially irreversible*. Strong fear responses may decrease to some extent with repeated nonreinforced exposures to the CS (with avoidance responses not permitted), but the fear will *never* go away completely according to these authors.

The unusual persistence of responses learned to avoid strong fear is very relevant to our understanding of neurotic disorder. Again two important factors are emphasized: classically conditioned fear does not extinguish readily even when avoidance responses are not permitted; and when anticipatory avoidance responses are learned that prevent the fear from being aroused, both the avoidance response and the fear become extremely persistent. By persistence of fear in the latter case, it is meant that, if at some future time the avoidance response is not made before presentation of the fear-eliciting stimulus, the fear response will recur.

MEDIATING STIMULI

It would be convenient if all conditioned stimuli and discriminative stimuli were external to the organism. Unfortunately this is not the case. There are many sources of stimuli within the organism that cannot be observed or readily controlled by an investigator, but which may serve as both conditioned stimuli and discriminative stimuli. There are visceral stimuli and probably stimuli that originate in more central parts of the nervous system associated with drive states such as hunger, thirst, sex, etc.; similar sources of stimuli associated with emotional reactions; and stimuli associated with all those higher thought processes that we subjectively know to exist— ideas, words, images, and fantasies. Expectations or beliefs of the form "in that situation this is likely to happen" or "if I do that, then such and such is likely to happen" may be especially potent as conditioned stimuli for emotional reactions or as discriminative stimuli for instrumental responses.

A nonobservable mediating conditioned stimulus is illustrated in a study by Miller (1951). First, subjects were conditioned to respond with a GSR to the letter T, spoken out loud, and *not* to the number 4, spoken out loud; The T's and 4's were presented in an unpredictable sequence and the subjects were given an electric shock every time they said T out loud. Then subjects were shown a series of dots and instructed to *think* T to the first one, 4 to the second, and so on alternately. Much larger GSR's occurred to the dots producing the thought of T than the dots producing the thought of 4.

Not only can these internal stimuli serve as conditioned and discriminative stimuli, they can also serve as dimensions of *stimulus generaliza-*

tion. The varied networks of associations based on similarities in meaning in human language provide a rich source of generalization stimuli. Generalization involving mediating language stimuli is frequently called semantic generalization. There is considerable evidence that autonomic responses conditioned to a specific word will generalize to other words of similar meaning. Lacey and Smith (1954) conditioned heart rate acceleration to the word "cow" and found generalization to other words with a rural meaning. Lang, Geer, and Hnatiow (1963) found similar words grouped according to four degrees of "hostile" meaning.

Experiments using discrete words as stimuli probably do not do justice to the complex channels of generalization available through internal thought processes—the meanings involved in sentences and larger language units, the nonlanguage stimuli associated with images or certain abstract concepts, and the various shadings of subjective emotion.

Visceral activity can also serve as conditioned stimuli for conditioned responses. Razran (1961) reviewed a number of studies by Russian researchers on this kind of conditioning. He described studies by Pogrebkova (1950, 1952) in which an intestinal loop was formed in five dogs so that an external source of air pressure could be introduced into the loop and produce rhythmic distentions (the CS). Air composed of 10% carbon dioxide was administered to the lungs and served as a UCS that produced increased respiration rate and general defensive reactions; the dogs learned to discriminate between intestinal distentions at a frequency of about 100 per minute and 15 per minute, responding to the 100 rate with increased respiratory activity and other signs of agitation. This conditioned response to the intestinal distention was reported to be highly resistant to extinction.

Results of this kind suggest the possibility that certain aspects of one emotional reaction can serve as conditioned stimuli for certain aspects of other emotional reactions. If fear reactions in a young child are followed by parent reactions that produce grief or shame, it is possible that in the future the child may respond to incipient fear reactions with grief or shame. The internal stimuli associated with fear now serve as conditioned stimuli eliciting the other emotional reactions. Thought processes may also help mediate such connections: "I am afraid. Only sissies are afraid and cowardly. I should be ashamed. . . ."

Not only can the stimuli associated with one emotion come to elicit another emotion, the stimuli from one emotion may come to serve as conditioned stimuli to elicit *more of the same* emotion. This seems to happen sometimes in the case of fear, when the pounding heart, trembling, fast breathing, etc., may serve as cues for more fear. Mediating thought processes probably also contribute to this. The person remembers how terrifying and generally upsetting past fear experiences have been and this thought serves as a stimulus for more fear. Or the person interprets the physical reactions in a way that leads to further fear, for example, that he is beginning to have a heart attack. Experimental investigation of this phenomenon is limited, but clinical observation strongly supports such a possibility.

OBSERVATIONAL LEARNING AND IMITATION

Imitation is an especially important phenomenon that cannot be explained readily by the principles of classical conditioning and instrumental learning. Bandura (1965a) reports an ingenious series of experiments demonstrating that children learn to make certain responses as a result of simply observing models making these responses. Since the child does not make the response before the test for learning, there is no easy way to argue that it has been reinforced. Bandura suggests that a learned association develops between a stimulus and a response on the basis of simultaneous sensory representations in the brain, and that no reinforcement is necessary. He does suggest, however, that whether a given response learned in this way will persist and become stronger is largely a function of the subsequent reinforcement history.

Imitation occurs for responses that are incidental or irrelevant to any obvious goals as well as for instrumental responses that the model uses to achieve some goal. Imitative learning probably plays an important role in the acquisition of language; behavioral traits of aggression, independence, sociability, etc.; and perhaps neurotic symptomatology. Especially important is the observational learning of reinforcement contingencies of the sort, "if a person does that, then such and such will happen," which can then come to serve as cognitive mediators that affect behavior. In this way a child may learn, for example, that it is safe or dangerous to do certain things, and his subsequent behavior will be controlled to some extent by these mediating thoughts.

Even classical conditioning of emotional responses can occur on the basis of observational learning. Bandura and Rosenthal (1966) and Berger (1962) have shown that young adult subjects, who observed other subjects supposedly being shocked and reacting with pain, responded with GSR's that became associated with conditioned stimuli. However, vicarious conditioning of this kind seems to necessitate some prior nonobservational conditioning in which the emotional responses of the subjects had become conditioned to the stimuli associated with administering shock, mediating cognitions about the painful effects of shock, or to another person's overt expressions of distress. More generally, vicarious conditioning seems to be based on the prior learning of empathic emotional responses to stimuli associated with another person's distress or to cognitions about the likely effects of certain experiences on another person in the absence of any direct observation of his distress; a person might have an empathic emotional response to simply being told that another person is going to receive a strong electric shock, even though he does not directly observe the other person's reaction.

Experimental studies have shown that imitation is enhanced if models are used that control sources of reinforcement for the child (Bandura, Ross, & Ross, 1963; Grusec, 1966; Grusec & Mischel, 1966; Mischel & Grusec, 1966) or if the child observes the model being reinforced for the behavior to be imitated (Bandura, 1965b; Bandura, Grusec, & Menlove, 1967; Walters & Parke, 1964).

Within the family, relative parent dominance appears to be an important factor in determining modeling influence. Hetherington (1965) found that normal children, age 4–11, tended to imitate the dominant parent in a standardized behavioral test situation regardless of sex of parent or sex of child. Parent dominance was determined from direct measures of parental interaction, such as which parent speaks first or last, passively accepts the other's suggestions, and talks the most. The influence of parent dominance on child imitative behavior may result from the greater salience of the dominant parent's behavior as well as the likelihood that the dominant parent controls more resources important to the child. It is also possible that the dominant parent is observed to "get his way" more often, and consequently be reinforced for his behavior.

CONFLICT

All human behavior continuously involves conflict and conflict resolution. The essential character of conflict is that two or more incompatible response tendencies are elicited by the same stimulus. There is nothing neurotic about the presence of conflict; it is an inescapable part of life. Most conflicts are resolved by simply opting for one response, by various compromise responses that maximize gains and minimize losses, or by escaping from the conflict situation. Certain kinds of conflict can, however, lead to behavioral and physiological indications of strong emotional reaction.

Experimental Neurosis in Animals

The now classical experiment by Shenger-Krestonvnikova reported by Pavlov (1928) has frequently been cited in support of the role of conflict in neurosis. A dog learned a conditioned discrimination so that he salivated in response to a circle but not to an ellipse. The ellipse was made more and more circular, until the dog could no longer make the discrimination. At this point the dog became "emotionally disturbed," began to struggle to escape from the experimental setting, to howl, and also lost the capacity to make appropriate conditioned salivary responses to differences in the stimuli that had previously been discriminated without difficulty.

A summary of procedures follows that have been found to produce emotional disturbance in dogs, cats, sheep, pigs, and rats.

1. Too difficult a discrimination between positive and negative CS or too rapid alternation between these stimuli. (Pavlov, 1928).

2. Continuous presentation of negative CS for too long a time period or discrete presentations at too high a frequency. (Pavlov, 1928; Anderson & Parmenter, 1941).

3. Monotonous repetition at regular intervals of positive CS reinforced by shock (Anderson & Parmenter, 1941; Liddell, 1956).

4. Pairing of aversive stimuli, such as shock or air blast, with consummatory responses such as eating (Liddell, 1956; Masserman, 1943).

There seems to be some element of conflict involved in all these procedures; either the animal is attempting to inhibit an inappropriate response to the negative CS under difficult circumstances or he tends to make a response to one discriminative stimulus that may result, unpredictably, in either positive reinforcement or an aversive consequence. On the other hand Wolpe (1958) and Smart (1965) found that presentations of the aversive stimuli alone, shock in this case, produced as much disturbance as presentations of the aversive stimuli paired with eating. Thus the role of conflict in procedure four needs additional study. An important feature in most of these procedures is that the animal cannot escape from the situation and is frequently physically restrained. It should be emphasized that within the same species some animals are more prone to show disturbances than others, and that the disturbance does not always generalize beyond the immediate experimental setting.

The disturbances are commonly of an excitatory kind in which the animal may show motor restlessness, trembling, low threshold of reaction and fast reaction times to external stimuli, howling, whining, other vocalizations, escape attempts, cardiac and respiratory acceleration or irregularity, increased frequency of urination and defecation, and vomiting. Less frequently the disturbance is inhibitory in nature and may involve immobility, falling asleep, and more rarely, cataleptic rigidity. Inherited differences in temperament may play an important role in determining disposition to excitatory or inhibitory reactions, although this has not been carefully investigated.

Following Gellhorn (1967) we would conclude that an important consequence so far as neurotic disorder is concerned is that procedures of this kind frequently result in a disturbance in the usual balance and level of activation in the hypothalamic systems, so that strong sympathetic responses alternate or occur simultaneously with strong parasympathetic responses, with resulting disruption of normal functioning, including the disruption of learned discriminations and other "higher" mental processes.

Conflict in Human Neurosis

It is questionable whether we should consider these "neurotic" disorders in animals as equivalent to neurotic disorders in humans. We shall not worry much about how these animal disturbances should be labeled; their value in the understanding of human neurotic disorder lies primarily in the suggestion that some of the same conditions that produce these emotional disturbances in animals may contribute to similar reactions in humans. In other words, they may suggest some hypotheses that would then have to be investigated with human subjects.

A kind of conflict that may be especially important in human neurotic disorder is that produced by the fourth animal procedure described above. This has been called an *approach-avoidance* conflict; the person has a tendency to both approach and avoid some goal object. This conflict is likely to be particularly distressing if both approach and avoidance tendencies are strong; the approach tendency is stronger than the avoidance tendency at points remote from the goal object, and the avoidance tendency is stronger than the approach tendency near the goal object; there is no escape from the conflict situation that would not be even more aversive than remaining. The aversiveness associated with escape might simply be the deprivation that would result from not obtaining the desired aspect of the goal.

The person caught in such a conflict may aptly be said to be "in a bind" or to have a "hang-up." He can neither approach nor avoid the goal completely and is likely to vacillate toward it and away from it at some intermediate distance. The college student who approaches a telephone to call a recently met girl for a date may alternately approach and retreat from the telephone as he anticipates the possibility of a new and enjoyable relationship on the one hand or rejection on the other. A child who has experienced both nurturance and punishment from his parents may likewise find himself in an approach-avoidance conflict.

SOCIAL LEARNING AND PERSONALITY DEVELOPMENT

The Interacting System

When learning is studied in the laboratory or certain structured educational settings, the learner has relatively little influence on the teacher or, in some cases, on the apparatus designed to give programmed instruction. The pace and level of difficulty of the presented materials may be varied as a function of the learner's progress but this is usually the limit of the learner's influence. In sharp contrast, most social learning situations involve two or more people where all parties influence each other, and there is no clear distinction between learner and teacher.

Consider a situation in which a six-month old infant cries when he awakens in the night. Its mother finds the crying aversive. She may verbalize this by saying she is afraid the infant is cold or sick, or that the infant will feel unloved and rejected if she does not comfort him, or that she simply cannot stand to hear her baby crying. At any rate she goes to the infant, holds it, and it stops crying. In this brief dyadic interaction both parties have made responses that were reinforced. The mother made the response of approaching and holding the infant, and was reinforced for this by the termination of an aversive stimulus, the crying. The infant made the response of crying, which was followed by the reinforcement of being held by the mother. Other things being equal, on similar future occasions both members of the dyad will have an even stronger tendency to repeat their respective responses. As a result the probability that this entire sequence of dyadic interaction will repeat itself has increased. In this example mother *and* infant are both teacher and learner.

A "systems" approach of this kind has implications for the cause and effect question. Assume that in the above example the interaction sequence has developed to such a point that at age 18 months mother is kept up half the night and cannot leave the infant with baby sitters because of the intensity of the crying-tantrum type behavior. Who has caused this unfortunate outcome? In the present moment it would seem that both cause it, since both reinforce the other for playing their respective roles in the interaction. In the more distant past one might say that mother caused it by responding to the infant's crying in the first place or perhaps by not stopping the response when the interaction sequence began to increase in strength. On the other hand the infant in the beginning may have been experiencing a period of real distress, colic for example, or an inherited tendency toward hyperactivity and "fussiness," that resulted in long periods of nightly crying to which the mother responded. The same mother might not have responded in the same way to the average amount of crying or "fussing" infants show before falling asleep or when they wake in the night. In that case we might say the infant caused the outcome.

It is a feature of interaction systems of this kind that after a while certain original causative factors may play no further role in the system. The original colic may no longer exist but the system continues as strong as ever. Another feature of systems such as this is a tendency to "escalate" to higher intensities and/or frequencies of occurrence, *providing other factors do not change.* The modification of such systems does not necessarily require that we understand the originating circumstances. When the system itself has generated highly aversive consequences for one or both participants, for the mother in this example, then other factors have changed and there is leverage for modifying the interaction sequence.

So far we have used dyadic (two-person) interaction as our model. The principles, however, apply to any number of interacting individuals. Obviously the analysis can get exceedingly complicated as we increase the number involved. Let us add father to the mother-infant pair to make a triad. Father may have been critical of mother, especially questioning her competence as a good mother. He may have been inclined to blame her for any little disturbance shown by the infant. She responds to this by over-responding to the infant's crying. Later when the mother-infant dyad is showing the greatly increased nightly crying, the father, not understanding the reinforcement contingencies producing it, may blame the mother for this too. She redoubles her efforts to be a good mother and inadvertently further reinforces the system.

Social interaction systems will vary in terms of how many people, or institutions, one must include in order to understand them. In some cases for all practical purposes it is not necessary to go beyond the dyad. In other cases complete understanding requires consideration of a third person, or an entire family plus grandparents, or even the religious institutions or sociological and economic conditions within which the family exists. Regardless, however, of how far we extend the system the actual implementation of the system must occur in terms of reinforcement contingencies acting upon individuals. For many purposes it may not be necessary to have complete understanding of all forces affecting a given system. In our example it might be that father does play an important role in maintaining the triadic interaction system but that the immediate influences of grandparents, the neighbors, the church, and society are relatively weak. Many of these sources may have played a past role in developing father's and mother's dispositions to behave in certain ways, and would be relevant to a complete historical account, but are not necessary to account for the current continuation of the system or to include in modification attempts.

Assessment

The data source. Ratings made from parent interviews or self-report questionnaires answered by parents have not paid off as an approach to the study of personality development. Yarrow, Campbell, and Burton (1968) and Becker and Krug (1965) summarize the disappointing results for the parent interview procedure and a well-known questionnaire, the Parent Attitude Research Instrument, respectively. Parent reports tend to be inconsistent over time (MacFarlane, 1938; Wenar, 1961) and show little agreement with reports by the spouse, children or extrafamilial sources (Becker, 1960; Goddard, Broder, & Wenar, 1961; Haggard, Brekstad, & Skard, 1960). These findings are not surprising if one considers the task that the parent is usually asked to perform. A mother, for example, is asked to recall past events (sometimes as much as 5–10 years previously), to rate herself on ambiguously defined features of child rearing, and to describe principles that guide her behavior with her child. In general this is a *weak* kind of data upon which to build a science of personality development.

Data based on direct observation of both child and parent is preferred, but this approach is not without problems. Such direct observation can range from naturalistic home observations to the use of highly structured tasks in the laboratory. The data will be valid only to the extent that these samples of interaction are indeed representative of significant family patterns and are not seriously distorted by the presence of observers. There is no easy road to the collection of good data in the study of personality development. It is probably advisable to assess family interaction by several avenues of measurement. In subsequent chapters I have given preference to studies that have made some use of direct observation.

Traits and situations. Another issue that is both conceptual and methodological involves the notion of traits. The term trait usually implies that an individual consistently manifests a given behavioral characteristic in a number of situations. A few individuals probably do show a high degree of consistency for a given behavior, but most individuals show a great deal of variation both in different situations and in the same situation on different occasions. For example, behavioral measures of conformity to moral standards in different situations have not been found to intercorrelate highly. Hartshorne and May (1928) exposed children to temptations to cheat, lie, and steal, and found some statistically significant correlations among measures, but the correlations were very low, averaging around .20. Sears et al. (1965) found little correlation between aggression observed in the nursery school, the laboratory, and in the home. Actually there have been few studies in which behavioral measures on such variables as dependency, aggression and anxiety were obtained in a variety of situations so that degree of generality could be evaluated. It seems likely that aggression will be found to be highly influenced by the target of the aggression and the situational context. Aggression may vary a great deal, for example, depending on whether the target is father, mother, brother, sister, teachers, male peers, or female peers. There is some evidence that preadolescent children tend to be consistent over time in rates of aggressive behavior if measures are obtained in the same general situation (Jersild & Markey, 1936; Kagan & Moss, 1962; Patterson, et al., 1967).

A related issue is the extent to which different kinds of behavior that are assumed to reflect one underlying trait actually intercorrelate with each other. For example, different behavioral measures of dependency (such as positive attention seeking, touching or holding, and seeking close physical proximity) have not been found to intercorrelate highly in young children (Heathers, 1953; Mann, 1959).

The implication of these findings is that our knowledge about personality development will rest on a firmer foundation if we specify both the situation and the specific nature of the response being measured, rather than uncritically assuming either situational generality or the equivalence of different types of responses.

Functional analysis. The kinds of assessment procedure that are likely to be useful, either for purposes of research or treatment, are those that emphasize a functional analysis of the discriminative stimuli and reinforcement contingencies that have produced and currently maintain the behavior of interest. Such an analysis would include careful description of the behavior being studied; the frequency, intensity or quickness of the behavior in different situations; the consequences that follow the behavior, categorized as reinforcing or punishing if possible; the presence of models for the behavior; mediating cognitions, inferred from self-reports, that affect the behavior; and information relevant to a systems analysis such as the consequences received by *other people* for responding in certain ways to the subject. Assessment information of this type might well provide a basis for diagnostic classification that would be much more useful than the traditional psychiatric categories.

Obviously, some behaviors and some consequences are more easily and objectively measured than others. Even when the reliability of measurement is relatively low, more useful information is likely to be obtained by following the strategy of a functional analysis than by turning to other measuring instruments that provide easily obtained but irrelevant measures. Assessment techniques based on the observation of social interaction in naturalistic settings or based on behavioral test situations designed to elicit relatively high frequencies of the target behavior are probably the best approaches. Information about mediating thought processes must, of course, be obtained from some form of self-report. Information obtained by interview, especially if focused on behavioral descriptions, can be useful in making functional analyses for purposes of clinical treatment, but should not be used as the *only* source of data for scientific research.

REFERENCES

Anderson, O. D., & Parmenter, R. A long-term study of the experimental neurosis in the sheep and in the dog. *Psychosom. Med. Monogr.*, 1941, **2**, Nos. 3 & 4.

Ax, A. F. The physiological differentiation between fear and anger in humans. *Psychosom. Med.*, 1953, **15**, 433–442.

Bandura, A. Vicarious processes: A case of no-trial learning. In L. Berkowitz (Ed.), *Advances in experimental social psychology* (Vol. 2). New York: Academic Press, 1965a, 1–55.

Bandura, A. Influence of models' reinforcement contingencies on the acquisition of imitative responses. *J. pers. soc. Psychol.*, 1965b, **1**, 589–595.

Bandura, A., Grusec, J. E., & Menlove, F. L. Some social determinants of self-monitoring reinforcement systems. *J. pers. soc. Psychol.*, 1967, **5**, 449–455.

Bandura, A. & Rosenthal, T. L. Vicarious classical conditioning as a function of arousal level. *J. pers. soc. Psychol.*, 1966, **3**, 54–62.

Bandura, A., Ross, D., & Ross, S. A. Imitation of film-mediated aggressive models. *J. abnorm. soc. Psychol.*, 1963, **66**, 3–11.

Becker, W. C. The relationship of factors in parental ratings of self and each other to the behavior of kindergarten children as rated by mothers, fathers, and teachers. *J. consult. Psychol.*, 1960, **24**, 507–527.

Becker, W. C., & Krug, R. S. The parent attitude research instrument—a research review. *Child Develop.*, 1965, **36**, 329–365.

Berger, S. M. Conditioning through vicarious instigation. *Psychol. Rev.*, 1962, **69**, 450–466.

Campbell, D., Sanderson, R. E., & Laverty, S. G. Characteristics of a conditioned response in human subjects during extinction trials following a single traumatic conditioning trial. *J. abnorm. soc. Psychol.*, 1964, **68**, 627–639.

Elder, T., Noblin, C. D., & Maher, B. A. The extinction of fear as a function of distance versus dissimilarity from the original conflict situation. *J. abnorm. soc. Psychol.*, 1961, **63**, 530–533.

Frankenhaeuser, M., Jarpe, G., Svan, H., & Wrangsjo, B. Physiological reactions to two different placebo treatments. *Scand. J. Psychol.*, 1963, **47**, 285–293.

Gellhorn, E. *Principles of Autonomic-Somatic Integrations.* Minneapolis: University of Minnesota Press, 1967.

Goddard, K. E., Broder, G., & Wenar, C. Special article—reliability of pediatric histories, a preliminary study. *Pediatrics*, 1961, **28**, No. 6.

Grusec, J. E. Some antecedents of self-criticism. *J. pers. soc. Psychol.*, 1966, **4**, 244–252.

Grusec, J. E., & Mischel, W. The model's characteristics as determinants of social learning. *J. pers. soc. Psychol.*, 1966, **4**, 211–215.

Haggard, E. A., Brekstad, A., & Skard, A. G. On the reliability of the anamnestic interview. *J. abnorm. soc. Psychol.*, 1960, **61**, 311–318.

Hartshorne, H., & May, M. A. *Studies in the Nature of Character. Vol. I. Studies in Deceit.* New York: Macmillan, 1928.

Hetherington, E. M. A developmental study of the effects of sex of the dominant parent on sex-role preference, identification, and imitation in children. *J. pers. soc. Psychol.,* 1965, **2,** 188–194.

Heathers, G. Emotional dependence and independence in a physical threat situation. *Child Develop.,* 1953, **24,** 169–179.

Hickham, J. B., Cargill, W. H., & Golden, G. Cardiovascular reactions to emotional stimuli: Effect on cardiac output, A-V oxygen difference, arterial pressure and peripheral resistance. *J. clin. Invest.,* 1948, **27,** 290–298.

Jersild, A. T., & Markey, F. V. Conflicts between pre-school children. *Child Develop. Monogr.,* 1935, No. 21.

Kagan, J., & Moss, H. A. *Birth to Maturity: A Study in Psychological Development.* New York: Wiley, 1962.

Kardiner, A. The neuroses of war. In S. S. Tomkins (Ed.), *Contemporary Psychopathology.* Cambridge: Harvard University Press, 1943.

Lacey, J. I., & Smith, R. L. Conditioning and generalization of unconscious anxiety. *Science,* 1954, **120,** 1045–1052.

Lang, P. J., Geer, J., & Hnatiow, M. Semantic generalization of conditioned autonomic responses. *J. exp. Psychol.,* 1963, **65,** 552–558.

Leopold, R. L., & Dillon, H. Psychoanatomy of a disaster: A long term study of post-traumatic neuroses in survivors of a marine explosion. *Amer. J. Psychiat.,* 1963, **119,** 913–921.

Liddell, H. S. *Emotional hazards in animals and man.* Springfield, Ill.: Charles C. Thomas, 1956.

Malmo, R. B., Boag, T. J., & Smith, A. A. Physiological study of personal interaction. *Psychosom. Med.,* 1957, **19,** 105–119.

Mann, R. D. A review of the relationships between personality and performance in small groups. *Psychol. Bull.,* 1959, **56,** 241–270.

Masserman, J. H. *Behavior and neurosis.* Chicago: University of Chicago Press, 1943.

MacFarlane, J. W. Studies in child guidance. I. Methodology of data collection and organization. *Mongr. society Res. Child Devlop.,* 1938, **3,** No. 6.

Miller, N. E. Learnable drives and rewards. In S. Stevens (Ed.), *Handbook of experimental psychology.* New York: Wiley, 1951.

Mischel, W., & Grusec, J. E. Determinants of the rehearsal and transmission of neutral and aversive behaviors. *J. pers. soc. Psychol.,* 1966, **3,** 197–205.

Mowrer, O. H. *Learning theory and personality dynamics.* New York: Ronald Press, 1950.

Olds, J. The central nervous system and the reinforcement of behavior. *Amer. Psychol.,* 1969, **24,** 114–132.

Patterson, G. R., Littman, R. A., & Bricker, W. Assertive behavior in children: A step towards a theory of aggression. *Monogr. soc. res. Child Develop.,* 1967.

Pavlov, I. P. *Lectures on conditioned reflexes.* (trans. W. H. Gantt) New York: International Publishers, 1928.

Pogrebkova, A. V. Conditioned reflexes to hypercapnia. *Dokl. Akad, Nauk* SSSR, 1950, **73,** 225–228.

Pogrebkova, A. V. Respiratory intero- and exteroceptive conditioned reflexes and their interrelationship. I: Formation and properties of respiratory intero- and exteroceptive conditioned reflexes. In K. M. Bykov (Ed.), *Voprosy fiziologii interotseptsii.* Moscow: Akad, Nauk SSSR, 1952.

Razran, G. The observable unconscious and the inferable conscious in current Soviet psychophysiology: Interoceptive conditioning, semantic conditioning, and the orienting reflex. *Psychol. Rev.,* 1961, **68,** 81–147.

Reich, W. *Character-analysis.* (trans. T. P. Wolfe) New York: Orgone Institute Press, 1949.

Sears, R. R., Rau, L., & Alpert, R. *Identification and Child Training.* Stanford, Calif.: Stanford University Press, 1965.

Shannon, I. L., Szmyd, L., & Prigmore, J. R. Stress in dental patients. *School of Aerospace Medicine Reports,* Brooks Air Force Base, Texas, 1962, No. 62–59, 6.

Smart, R. G. Effects of alcohol on conflict and avoidance behavior. *Quart. Journal of Studies on Alcohol,* 1965, **26,** 187–205.

Solomon, R. L. Kamin, L. J., & Wynne, L. C. Traumatic avoidance learning: The outcomes of several extinction procedures with dogs. *J. abnorm. soc. Psychol.,* 1953, **48,** 291–302.

Solomon, R. L. & Wynne, L. C. Traumatic avoidance learning: The principles of anxiety conservation and partial irreversibility. *Psychol. Rev.,* 1954 **61,** 353–385.

Walters, R. H., & Parke, R. D. Influence of response consequences to a social model on resistance to deviation. *J. exper. Child Psychol.,* 1964, **1,** 269–280.

Watson, J. B., & Rayner, R. Conditioned emotional reactions. *J. exp. Psychol.,* 1920, **3,** 1–14.

Wenar, C. The reliability of mother's histories. *Child Develop.,* 1961, **32,** 491–500.

Wolpe, J. *Psychotherapy by reciprocal inhibition.* Stanford, Calif.: Stanford University Press, 1958.

Yarrow, M. R., Campbell, J. D., & Burton, R. V. *Child rearing: An inquiry into research and methods.* San Francisco: Jossey-Bass, 1968.

CHAPTER SIX

LEARNED AVOIDANCE
STRATEGIES

Concepts derived from basic research on learning processes will now be applied to an important feature of many neurotic disorders, the avoidance of aversive consequences. Because this book is primarily concerned with neurotic disorder, constructive and nonneurotic modes of coping with aversive consequences will not be emphasized. These would be important to consider in any comprehensive analysis of personality development. In general, actions aimed at attacking or modifying the basic conditions responsible for the aversive consequences would be of this kind. There are no sharp lines, however, between constructive, nonneurotic coping responses and the avoidance responses to be discussed below. We all employ avoidance responses to some extent, and they should be considered part of a neurotic pattern only if they result in extreme interference in normal patterns of living. Somewhat arbitrarily, avoidance responses are divided into those that consist of overt or observable behavior and those that are covert and must be inferred from other responses.

OVERT RESPONSES

Physical Avoidance

This response is so obvious as to need little elucidation. The person simply removes himself physically from those stimuli that produce aversive consequences. It may involve no more than turning one's head away from or closing one's eyes to an unpleasant sight—an accident, or a scary movie, for example. Or it may involve more complete physical avoidance: one does not make public speeches, climb steep mountains, go to social gatherings, or make a date with a girl. This type of avoidance response can only work with external stimuli. Obviously one cannot physically avoid internal thoughts and drive states.

Physical avoidance is probably one of the most commonly used avoidance responses. Extremes of social withdrawal or avoidance of certain situations or objects are seen in the phobic reactions.

Displacement

The displacement phenomenon can best be understood in terms of generalization gradients associated with an approach-avoidance conflict, *when certain other avenues of response are available.* Murray and Berkun (1955) provided a demonstration of stimulus displacement using rats in three parallel alleys with removable doorways between alleys. Using food and shock, an approach-avoidance conflict was established in one of the side alleys, with entrances to the other alleys closed. The doors to the other alleys were then opened. Rats did indeed displace their approach responses to the other alleys. The farther they got away from the original alley, the nearer they moved to the goal.

Displacement can also occur along a dimension of response similarity. Thus a strong urge to physically attack another person might be displaced by some kind of verbal attack.

There has been surprisingly little experimental research on displacement in humans. Kaufman and Feshbach (1963) found that subjects who were angered by gratuitous insults given by an experimenter proposed more severe punishments for a juvenile delinquent than did subjects who were not previously insulted. Murray (1954) provides quantitative data from psychotherapy interviews that suggest that the patient "approached" the direct expression of verbal aggression toward his mother in the same fashion as the rats in the other study had "approached" the food boxes in the alleys: tentatively, over the course of 17 interviews, after some initial mild aggressive expression toward his mother, the patient turned to aggressive expression toward his aunt, then toward other people, and then near the end returned to express aggression more directly toward his mother.

Use of Positive Affect to Reduce Negative Affect

The effectiveness of this strategy is intuitively obvious. A young child who sucks his thumb or holds his "security" blanket against his face when distressed exemplifies the basic principle. Watson and Rayner (1920) report the anecdotal observation that after conditioning, Albert engaged in more thumb sucking when furry objects were present than when not present. The principle of inducing positive affect to reduce negative affect has, in fact, been developed into *systematic desensitization,* a major treatment technique for anxiety reactions.

The variations on this strategy are limited only by the types of positive-affect-inducing procedures available to people. Alcohol and other drugs, tobacco smoking, sex, and food can be used in this way. This is not to say that these activities cannot be engaged in as ends in themselves, that is, for the sake of the positive enjoyment alone. They can be. The point here is that they can *also* serve the purpose of negative affect reduction. When these activities do serve the purpose of reduction of strong negative affect, they take on a compulsive quality, by which it is meant that they are highly persistent even in the face of secondary aversive consequences. Thus, a person may persist with compulsive masturbation even though he subsequently feels remorse, or with compulsive eating even though he is overweight, or with compulsive drinking even though he subsequently becomes physically ill or encounters social difficulties.

The excitement and exhilaration associated with certain moderately dangerous activities such as sports car racing, parachute jumping, or even riding a roller coaster can serve this kind of purpose. Of course the thrills (positive affect) involved in such activities can have various sources, the successful mastery of danger, the physical sensations, or the acclaim of an audience or peer group. The simple presence of other people is anxiety reducing for some individuals. Schachter (1959), for example, found that some college students preferred to wait with other students rather than alone when anticipating a stressful experience.

The emotion of anger, if not especially positive, may be at least considerably less negative than fear, and thus serve to reduce the negative affect of fear. In other words, some individuals may learn to become angry when confronted with fear-arousing stimuli as a way of controlling the magnitude of fear aroused. Recall the greater g tolerance of subjects who reacted aggressively in the centrifuge compared to those who reacted with anxiety (p. 39). The evidence that individuals may learn to be angry in order to reduce anxiety is only suggestive, but it is a reasonable hypothesis at this time.

The use of positive affect to reduce negative affect assumes some degree of incompatibility between the responses involved. Processes of reciprocal inhibition in the hypothalamic autonomic systems may be involved. There is always a possibility that the negative affect is so intense that instead of being inhibited by the positive affect it becomes conditioned to the stimuli associated with the positive affect. For example, instead of the positive affect associated with eating coming to inhibit anxiety, stimuli associated with eating may come to elicit more anxiety.

The use of positive affect to reduce negative affect is seen most clearly in disorders not usually labeled neurotic, such as antisocial behavior, sexual deviation, and drug addiction. It does occur, however, as part of the larger pattern in many neurotic disorders, and its role should not be minimized.

Behavioral Traits

Individuals sometimes develop behavioral traits or whole styles of life that are largely based on negative affect avoidance. Traits of passivity or femininity in men may reflect an attempt to avoid assertive, competitive, or aggressive responses toward other men because of fears of counterattack. Extreme traits of courteousness, politeness, formality, pedantry, orderliness, or nonemotionality may serve similarly as avoidance strategies. The term *reaction formation* has been used to refer to traits that seem primarily oriented toward preventing an expression of an opposite tendency, for example, passive-submissive instead of aggressive-competitive tendencies. Reich (1949) has used the term *character armor* to aptly describe such traits, and provides a number of clinical examples from his psychoanalytic practice.

Sanford (1942) made an extensive quantitative analysis of speech styles in two college students. The speech of one of these students was characterized by the following: 1) complexity, involving many intricately connected clauses; 2) frequent repetitions and rephrasings; 3) thoroughness, leaving out nothing that was remotely relevant; 4) many hesitations, uh's and ah's; 5) cautious wording, many qualifications, including frequent use of phrases such as "seems to be," or "might." Sanford summarized the speaking style as one reflecting a desire to avoid blame or disapproval by being cautious and indirect. A more intensive personality study of the same individual by White (1963) indicated that the speech characteristics were part of a larger pattern of behavioral traits oriented toward blame avoidance.

COVERT RESPONSES

The "Not-Think-About-It" Response

The avoidance response involved here is similar, and perhaps the same, as the mechanism of repression described by Freud and used as an important explanatory concept within psychoanalytic theory. Freud and his followers deserve credit for the explication of this mechanism and the wealth of examples of its operation provided in the clinical literature. It is reasonable to accept the proposal of Freud that some people will simply stop thinking about an experience that has been highly unpleasant, and thus avoid re-arousing the unpleasant memory. Some soldiers who have had terrifying combat experiences seem to engage in similar "not-think-about-it" strategies to avoid reactivation of the painful memory. For World War I see Kardiner (1943) and for World War II see Grinker and Spiegel (1945). The term repression will not be exphasized because, as used within the context of psychoanalytic theory, it tends to carry along additional meanings involving the unconscious, instinctual impulses, ego, superego, id, stages of psychosexual development, and other concepts that should not be introduced uncritically into the formulations. The "not-think-about-it" response is conceived simply as a kind of avoidance response involving covert thought processes. It may be more correct to label it a "think-about-something-else" response since the person probably does that rather than think about nothing at all.

Investigators have attempted to experimentally study repression but with only limited success, at least as far as convincing psychoanalytic practitioners that the research really had much to do with the concept as defined within their theory. A study that comes close to demonstrating the mechanism as defined here is that of Eriksen and Kuethe (1956). Their research used overt verbal responses, but it is reasonable to assume that covert thoughts could function in a similar fashion. They presented subjects with a series of 15 stimulus words one at a time, and told them to respond with the first word that came to mind. Prior to the experiment five of the words had been designated as "critical" stimuli. During the first presentation of the 15-word series the subject's responses to these five words were accompanied by a strong electric shock. Without pause the series was presented again and again, and every time the original response to one of the five critical stimulus words was given, the subject was shocked. The position of the critical stimulus words in the series was varied from trial to trial.

The purpose of the study was to see if subjects would learn, with or without awareness, to replace the shocked response with another response. In order to maximize the opportunity for "learning without awareness" subjects were misinformed as to the nature of the experiment. They were told that shocks would occur under two conditions: (1) if their response to a stimulus word was too slow for that particular stage of practice and (2) a second condition that could not be divulged in advance, but one that they might discover on their own and thus avoid receiving shocks.

After the procedure had been administered, the subjects were interviewed to ascertain degree of awareness of the real basis of the shocks.

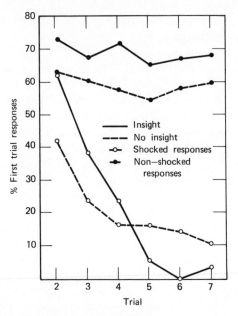

FIGURE 7.   Percentage of first-trial responses repeated on succeeding trials as a function of punishment (Eriksen & Kuethe, 1956).

Eleven high-awareness subjects were able to describe the real basis for the shocks and say what they had done to avoid them. All reported withholding punished responses while trying to think of another response to substitute for it, but that after a few trials it was no longer necessary to deliberately withhold the punished response since the new response began to occur "automatically." Another 11 subjects were classified as having low awareness. They were either unable to state any reason or gave wrong reasons for the basis of the shock. Nine subjects either had partial insight or were otherwise unclassifiable and results on these subjects were not reported.

Avoidance learning curves are shown in Figure 7. It can be seen that both aware and nonaware groups learned to avoid making the shocked response. The apparent differences in the learning curves were not statistically significant. Measures of time to give a response following presentation of the stimulus word, reaction times, were also obtained and curves for this measure are shown in Figure 8. The interesting feature in these curves is the initial increase in reaction time for the aware group, corroborating their subsequent report that they had searched for a substitute word in the early trials before the new response became "automatic." The nonaware group seems to have learned to substitute a new word without going through this intermediate stage.

There results suggest an analogy to learning certain motor skills such as typewriting. In the early stages of such learning a person is likely to be aware of the processes involved in associating a certain letter with a certain finger movement. As learning proceeds the responses become much more "automatic" and the person becomes able to type rapidly "without awareness" or without thinking about the individual finger movements. In the early stages of learning to not think about certain things associated with strong negative affect the person might well be aware to some extent of the connection between the stimulus ideas and the resulting negative affect. As learning proceeds, however, the "think-about-something else" response is made with increasingly shorter latencies (reaction times) and becomes more "automatic." It begins to serve as a true avoidance response in that the negative affect is almost completely avoided. This is especially true where similar stimuli, perhaps along dimensions of semantic similar-

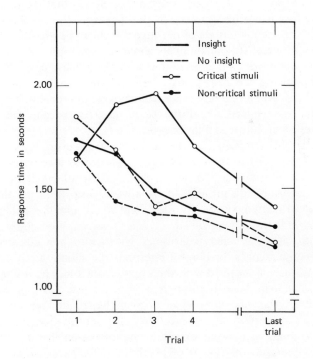

FIGURE 8. Reaction times to critical and noncritical stimuli as a function of trials (Eriksen & Juethe, 1956).

ity, come to serve as discriminative stimuli that elicit the "think-about-something-else" response before the critical stimuli even occur.

A variation on the "think-about-something-else" response is to think about things that produce positive affect. This is, of course, the same strategy described in the earlier section on overt responses, except that in this case no overt action is involved. Daydreaming can serve this function, that is, the avoidance of negative affect by daydreaming about pleasurable subjects that produce positive affect. Again all daydreaming of this kind does not necessarily serve to inhibit negative affect, but it can serve this purpose.

Cognitive Interpretations

The avoidance strategies to be discussed in this section primarily involve beliefs or interpretations. The essential idea is that the degree of aversiveness associated with a particular situation can be influenced by what one believes about the situation. If, while walking down a lonely street at night, one believes that he is likely to be attacked and robbed, fear is a probable response. If a person confidently believes that there is no danger of attack, fear is not likely to occur. In other words, given the same objective situation, the magnitude of negative affect can be greatly influenced by what we tell ourselves, our thoughts about the situation. Terms such as beliefs, interpretations, and expectations all refer to these covert thought processes. Following the paradigms of escape and avoidance learning, it is suggested that when one makes a certain covert interpretive response, negative affect is reduced, the response is thus reinforced, and it is more likely to occur in future similar occasions.

Beliefs that represent extreme deviations from everyday social consensus and that persist in the face of clear evidence to the contrary would be classified as delusions and are more characteristic of psychotic rather than neurotic levels of disturbance. Less severe distortions in thinking are prominent in many neurotic disorders, and we assume that ordinary escape or avoidance learning is involved.

Denial. When a person confronted with a situation that may result in aversive consequences for himself interprets the situation in a way that *denies* the features associated with the aversive outcome, he is employing the denial mechanism. Usually the person does not just deny some unpleasant truth, but asserts some contrary or opposite belief. For normal or neurotic individuals to employ denial effectively, the information must be incomplete or ambiguous to some extent. If the unpleasant truth is based on incontrovertible fact, then short of psychotic delusion, a person simply has to believe it. He may employ other negative affect reducing strategies such as not thinking about it, but he cannot deny the reality. A patient dying of cancer may interpret his illness in terms of some nonfatal disease and thus reduce the fear that he might have at the prospect of death. He may not have received from physicians and family members strong proof of the likely fatal outcome, and there is leeway for other beliefs about his illness.

Another common source of reinforcement for denying unpleasant outcomes, in this example as well as others, comes from the social environment. The people surrounding a dying patient, especially family members, but also the hospital staff, are uncomfortable about the prospect of death and are likely to join in what might be called a denial conspiracy in which any admission of the hopeless condition is avoided, and unfounded reassurances about recovery are used to reinforce the patient's false beliefs. The patient, in fact, may find himself now confronted with another source of negative affect, the discomfort and withdrawal of those close to him if he does not pretend along with them that everything will be all right. Under these circumstances it may be difficult to know to what extent the patient *really* believes the denial as opposed to verbalizing denial in order to retain a relationship with those close to him. Hackett and Weisman (1962) report findings similar to these in a clinical study of patients' and relatives' reactions to the prospect of imminent death.

Janis (1958) reported a clinical study of patients before and after surgery. Patients were rated in terms of the extent to which they showed preoperative fear associated with the dangers and discomforts associated with the operation. Patients who showed the least preoperative fear frequently denied certain realistic expectations about the postoperative discomfort involved and considered the surgeons to be infallible in their skills. These patients with the strong denial tendencies showed the greatest disturbance after surgery, involving anger and disappointment when denial of the realities was no longer possible. Janis' study points up the necessity for some degree of informational ambiguity in order for the denying belief to work, and that when reality becomes inescapable, as was the case after surgery, the avoidance strategy fails. It is of interest to note that the patients who expressed moderate degrees of preoperative fear showed the least psychological disturbance postoperatively.

Several studies report low physiological arousal accompanying the use of denial, suggesting that the denial mechanism is indeed serving its aim of negative affect reduction. Price et al. (1957) studied a group of patients facing thoracic or cardiac surgery. They found that patients rated as successfully employing defenses had lower levels of adrenocortical hormones in blood samples than those whose defenses were not successful. Defenses in this study seemed largely to involve denial of dangers involved in the surgery. Friedman et al. (1963) studied a group of husbands and wives whose children were stricken with incurable cancer. Most of these parents showed increases in urinary products of adrenocortical hormones during periods of more acute stress such as cardiac arrest, unexpected massive hemorrhage, or the death of the child. The authors selected the two fathers and two mothers who were considered as most effectively employing defensive mechanisms. Again the defenses seemed to largely involve denial as the following quotation suggests: "A father angrily insisted with each successive drug that was used on his child that it would be 'the cure' and would spend many hours verbalizing pseudomedical support for this contention. Another father told all of his friends that the doctors had 're-versed the diagnosis of leukemia' in his child (which unfortunately was not a correct statement) and then felt reassured when they expressed their happiness over his good news. One mother became angry with the other parents when they discussed the grave prognosis of leukemia, insisting that she would 'proceed with making college plans' for her child." (1963, pp. 374—375).

The average level of urinary indices of adrenocortical hormones was lower for the parents using these rather extreme denial defenses than the average for all the other parents. In a subsequent analysis of the data using the total sample of parents, Wolff et al. (1964) were able to predict considerably better than chance what the urinary indices would be from a knowledge of the effectiveness of parent defenses.

The above studies are correlational in nature and the direction of cause and effect is indeterminate. Rather than denial resulting in less negative affect, it may be that individuals who react with less negative affect to begin with can more readily use denial defenses. Several studies involving experimental manipulation of the denial response provide stronger evidence for its effectiveness in reducing physiological behavioral, and self-report components of emotional arousal.

Modifying the effects of drugs and placebos by creating different beliefs or expectations about their effects is an example of such experimental manipulation. For example, Frankenhaeuser et al. (1963) gave white or pink capsules to subjects on two different occasions. Both capsules were inert placebos. The white capsule was described to the subjects as a sleeping pill, the pink capsule as a stimulant. This experimental manipulation of beliefs about the same placebo (except for color) had definite and opposite effects on the subjects' self-reports of alertness, speed on a reaction-speed test, and also affected heart rate and blood pressure.

Schachter and Singer (1962) and Schachter and Wheeler (1962) have also demonstrated the role of cognitive interpretations in influencing emotional reactions. In the former study subjects were given epinephrine injections and observed a stooge modeling either euphoria or anger. Subjects who were not informed about the true nature of the physiological effects of epinephrine were highly influenced by a stooge and expressed whichever emotion he manifested. Subjects who were given correct information about what to expect from the epinephrine injections were less influenced by the stooge. The authors theorized that some degree of general physiological arousal is necessary for an emotional experience but the specific form of the emotion, that is, whether anger, euphoria, fear, or grief depends largely on the cognitive interpretation placed on the arousal. And these cognitive interpretations are highly affected by external circumstances.

To further explore this theory, Schachter and Wheeler (1952) administered epinephrine, placebo, and chlorpromazine (a tranquilizer that inhibits sympathetic arousal) to three groups of subjects without giving information about expected physiological effects. Measures of amusement or laughter to an excerpt from a comedy film were then obtained. As predicted, amusement expression was highest for epinephrine, next for placebo, and lowest for chlorpromazine. The authors take these findings as support for the notion that some degree of general physiological arousal is a necessary but not a sufficient condition to produce a specific emotional reaction. In addition a cognitive interpretation must be applied to the general arousal state.

The mechanism referred to as rationalization can be seen as a type of denial. This cognitive maneuver is familiar to all of us. The fox in Aesop's fable that decided the unreachable grapes were probably sour is a well-known example. The basic strategy is to change a belief or evaluation of events in order to reduce associated aversiveness.

Festinger (1957) has attempted to explain the "sour grapes" phenomenon in terms of conflicting or dissonant cognitions. He has proposed that whenever a person experiences two conflicting cognitions (beliefs, attitudes, opinions, etc.) he will tend to modify one of these cognitions so as to reduce the dissonance. Festinger and his colleagues have published many experiments demonstrating that people tend to change beliefs in order to reconcile conflicting points of view. The results of most of these studies can, perhaps, be just as readily interpreted in terms of *aversiveness reduction* as some need to reduce cognitive conflicts per se. In the case of the sour grapes, for example, it is probably not some universal need to reduce conflicting cognitions, but the negative affect associated with the continuation of unrequited need that is reduced by denial of the belief that the grapes are sweet and assertion of the new belief that the grapes are sour.

Intellectualization. Intellectualization may not be the best label to use for the class of avoidance techniques to be discussed here, but it has a tradition of usage and we will stick with it. The surgeon who cuts people open, the male physician who intimately examines unclothed women, the undertaker who prepares bodies for burial, and the general who issues the order that will certainly mean death or horrible injury to thousands of his soldiers—all of these individuals must somehow learn to avoid or minimize the strong emotional reactions that would ordinarily accompany these actions. If they do not learn to inhibit them, the resulting emotional reactions would seriously interfere with their performance. Part of the meaning of the word "professional" involves this very thing, the capacity to remain calm and unemotional in the carrying out of one's job—not to "lose one's cool." *Isolation* is a term that has also been used to refer to this "separation" of thoughts and behavior from emotional reaction.

Perhaps this capacity is not altogether a cognitive or interpretive process. It may partly involve the learning of some more direct noncognitive response that serves to inhibit emotional response. Or it may turn out to be a variant on the "think-about-something-else" response in which the something else is professional, task-oriented thoughts. The surgeon directs his full attention to the technical aspects of the operation, the general to the details of strategy and tactics, etc. It differs, however, from the type of "think-about-something-else" response described earlier in that the person does not stop thinking about the central subject matter, but rather changes the way in which he thinks about it. And most importantly, he probably prevents the chaining of associations that might produce continuing increase in emotion—the general brooding about the suffering of his soldiers and their relatives, the physician elaborating erotic fantasies about his unclothed female patient, and so on.

A provocative series of experiments by Lazarus and his colleagues indicates that intellectualization as well as denial can reduce negative affect. In an early study, Lazarus et al. (1962) showed that the presentation of a stressful film in the laboratory produced higher levels of skin conductance and heart rate than a nonstressful control film. Furthermore, increases in the two autonomic measures paralleled the several points of acute stress in the film. The stressful film, entitled *Subincision,* depicts a ceremony of an aboriginal Australian tribe in which a sequence of crude operations are performed on the penis and scrotum of adolescent boys. The nonstressful film was entitled *Corn Farming in Iowa.*

Speisman et al. (1964) used the same film, *Subincision,* as a stressor, but showed it under four experimental conditions: 1) silent, without sound track; 2) trauma; 3) denial and reaction formation; and 4) intellectualization. These conditions were implemented by sound track commentaries that accompanied the film. In the trauma condition the commentary emphasized the pain, cruelty, danger, and primitiveness of the rites. In the denial and reaction formation condition, the harmful aspects were denied (for example, by saying that the operation was not painful), and the positive benefits of participation in the ritual were emphasized by describing it as a joyful occasion for the native boys who looked forward with enthusiasm to becoming adult members of the tribe. In the intellectualization condition a scientific attitude toward the ritual was encouraged. The viewer was asked to observe the film in a detached manner, as anthropologists might, analyzing the interesting customs of the primitive natives. Fifty-six college students were assigned randomly to the four experimental conditions.

Skin conductance was highest under the trauma condition, next highest in the denial condition, the lowest in the intellectualization condition. It was significantly lower under both the denial and intellectualization conditions than the silent condition. Similar trends occurred for heart rate, but they were not statistically significant for certain comparisons.

Lazarus and Alfert (1964) performed a similar experiment in which they found that denial instructions preceding a silent presentation of the film were just as effective in reducing skin conductance and heart rate as the denial commentary accompanying the film. To further verify the results of these studies and to test the generality of results when a different kind of stressor film was used, Lazarus et al. (1965) performed the following experiment. College students were randomly assigned to the following three conditions: 1) control, 2) denial, and 3) intellectualization. An industrial safety film which portrayed three shop accidents was used as stressor. First, a worker lacerates a finger. Second, another worker amputates a finger in a milling machine. Third, a circular saw drives a board through the abdomen of a worker, who dies, writhing and bleeding on the floor.

The different experimental conditions were created prior to showing the film. In the denial condition the subjects were instructed to remember that the people in the film were actors and that none of them were actually injured. This theme was elaborated on by telling them, for example, that in order to give the impression of bleeding, red dye was squeezed from the palm of the hand. In the intellectualization condition the emphasis was on analyzing the technique used in the film to promote industrial safety. The subjects were urged to consider the sociopsychological factors involved when a shop foreman attempts to promote shop safety. No attempt was made to provide cognitive defenses in the control group.

The results for skin conductance are shown in Figure 9. The results generally confirm those of previous experiments with both denial and intellectualization showing less autonomic arousal than the control condition. Heart rate showed similar trends.

In viewing these experiments by Lazarus and his colleagues it seems reasonable to conclude that autonomic responses to stressful films can be reduced by the kinds of cognitive strategy that the authors label denial and intellectualization. Although not all comparisons between the "defense"

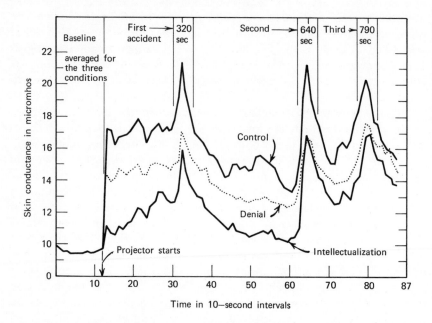

FIGURE 9. Effects of the experimental conditions on skin conductance (baselines equalized by covariance adjustment) (Lazarus, Opton, Nomikos, & Rankin, 1965).

conditions and the control conditions reached the .05 level of statistical significance, there seems to be enough consistency of results across independent samples of subjects in the various studies to warrant this conclusion.

The phenomenon of depersonalization may involve an extreme manifestation of the intellectualization response, or it may involve a more primitive and noncognitive avoidance strategy. Depersonalization as described by self-report involves the experience that one's surroundings, sometimes including oneself, are not real. The person experiences everything in a detached way as though he were an external observer calmly watching himself. Lader and Wing (1964), in their study of habituation in anxiety-reaction patients, describe a depersonalization episode.

"The patient, a woman, appeared fairly anxious before the test, and for the first two-thirds of the recording session the trace obtained was very active with a low skin resistance (high conductance), many fluctuations and persisting responses to stimuli. The activity increased and then, fairly suddenly, it decreased; the skin resistance soared upwards, the fluctuations diminished greatly in number and the responses habituated almost to zero. On questioning the patient afterwards, she reported that she felt a panic attack coming on about two-thirds of the way through the session. The feeling of panic increased until she felt that she would have to ask for the recording to be stopped. However, the feeling of panic suddenly subsided, and instead she felt that her surroundings were no longer real, that the walls of the room had disappeared, and that there were no recording electrodes attached to her arm." (p. 215)

CONCLUDING COMMENTS

People employ an infinite variety of strategies in coping with life's aversiveness. The ones we have discussed represent more common classes of these strategies, and in some cases ones which have been studied systematically. Much of the variety of neurotic symptomatology can be attributed to this diversity in learned strategies of avoidance.

REFERENCES

Eriksen, C. W., & Kuethe, J. L. Avoidance conditioning of verbal behavior without awareness: A paradigm of repression. *J. abnorm. soc. Psychol.*, 1956, **53**, 203–209.

Festinger, L. *A Theory of Cognitive Dissonance.* Stanford, Calif.: Stanford Univer. Press, 1957.

Frankenhaeuser, M., Jarpe, G., Svan, H., & Wrangsjo, B. Physiological reactions to two different placebo treatments. *Scand. J. Psychol.*, 1963, **47**, 285–293.

Friedman, S. B., Mason, J. W., & Hamburg, D. A. Urinary 17-hydroxycorticosteriod levels in parents of children with neoplastic disease: a study of chronic psychological stress. *Psychosom. Med.*, 1963, **25**, 364–376.

Grinker, R. R., & Spiegel, J. P. *Men under stress.* New York: McGraw Hill Book Company, 1945.

Hackett, T. P. & Weisman, A. D. Reactions to the imminence of death. In G. H. Grosser, H. Wechsler, & M. Greenblat (Eds.), *The threat of impending disaster.* Cambridge, Mass.: M.I.T. Press, 1964.

Janis, I. L. *Psychological stress.* New York: John Wiley & Sons, Inc., 1958.

Kardiner, A. The neuroses of war. In S. S. Tomkins (Ed.), *Contemporary Psychopathology.* Cambridge: Harvard Univer. Press, 1943.

Kaufman, H., & Feshbach, S. Displaced aggression and its modification through exposure to antiaggressive communications. *J. abnorm. soc. Psychol.*, 1963, **67**, 79–83.

Lader, M. H., & Wing, Lorna. Habituation of the psycho-galvanic reflex in patients with anxiety states and in normal subjects. *J. neurol., neurosurg., Psychiat.,* 1964, **27,** 210–218.

Lazarus, R. S., & Alfert, Elizabeth. Short-circuiting of threat by experimentally altering cognitive appraisal. *J. abnorm. soc. Psychol.,* 1964, **69,** 195–205.

Lazarus, R. S., Opton, E. M., Nomikos, M. S., & Rankin, N. O. The principle of short-circuiting of threat: further evidence. J. Pers., 1965, **33,** 622–635.

Lazarus, R. S., Speisman, J. C., Mordkoff, A. M., & Davison, L. A. A laboratory study of psychological stress produced by a motion picture film. *Psychol. Monogr.,* 1962, **76,** No. 34 (Whole No. 553).

Murray, E. J. A case study in a behavioral analysis of psychotherapy. *J. abnorm. soc. Psychol.,* 1954, **49,** 305–310.

Murray, E. J., & Berkun, M. M. Displacement as a function of conflict. *J. abnorm. soc. Psychol.,* 1955, **51,** 47–56.

Price, D. B., Thaler, M., & Mason, J. W. Preoperative emotional states and adrenal cortical activity. *AMA Arch. neurol. Psychiat.,* 1957, **77,** 646–656.

Sanford, F. H. Speech and personality: A comparative case study. *Char. & Pers.,* 1942, **10,** 169–198.

Schachter, S. *The psychology of affiliation.* Stanford, Calif.: Stanford Univer. Press, 1959.

Schachter, S., & Singer, J. E. Cognitive, social, and physiological determinants of emotional state. *Psychol. Rev.,* 1962, **69,** 379–399.

Schachter, S., & Wheeler, L. Epinephrine, chlorpromazine, and amusement. *J. abnorm. soc. Psychol.,* 1962, **65,** 121–128.

Speisman, J. C., Lazarus, R. S., Mordkoff, A. M., & Davison, L. A. Experimental reduction of stress based on ego-defense theory. *J. abnorm. soc. Psychol.,* 1964, **68,** 367–380.

Watson, J. B., & Rayner, R. Conditioned emotional reactions. *J. exp. Psychol.,* 1920, **3,** 1–14.

Wolff, C. T., Friedman, S. B. Hofer, M. A., & Mason, J. W. Relationship between psychological defenses and mean urinary 17-hydroxycorticosteroid excretion rates: I. A predictive study of parents of fatally ill children. *Psychosom. Med.,* 1964, **26,** 576–591.

CHAPTER SEVEN

DEVELOPMENT: GENERAL FEATURES OF NEUROTIC DISORDER

There have been many theories about the development of neurotic disorders. Historically the theories of Freud have been influential, and a brief and oversimplified outline of the Freudian theory of neurosis is presented in this section.

Personality development centers around biologically determined stages of psychosexual development in which the basic sexual instinct (the libido) seeks gratification via oral, anal, and, finally, genital zones of the body. Fixation and regression to these various stages of development influence later personality traits, including features of neurotic symptomatology. In the Freudian theory of neurosis anxiety plays a central role, especially anxiety associated with an unresolved oedipal conflict. The oedipal conflict is an assumed inevitable sexual attraction that a young child will have toward the opposite sex parent and the resulting competition with, and fear of, the same sex parent. In boys, for example, irrational fantasies involving death wishes toward the father and expected retaliation in the form of castration are thought to be the basis for most neurotic anxieties. The oedipal conflict becomes most intense when the child is 4–6 years of age, and in an effort to reduce the associated anxiety the entire conflict is repressed at that time.

The adult anxiety reaction is thought to represent the "breaking through" of the "dammed up" anxiety without awareness of the childhood oedipal conflict that gave rise to the anxiety. The phobic reaction is considered to have a similar origin except that in addition to the original repression of the oedipal conflict, the anxiety is said to be displaced from its initial source (fear of castration by father in boys) to the external phobic situation. This is considered to be a defense or avoidance strategy because the external situation is easier to avoid than internal thoughts about castration or the external presence of father. Many of the symptoms seen in the obsessive compulsive and hysterical disorders are considered to be defenses or avoidance strategies aimed at keeping the oedipal conflict and its associated anxiety under control.

Neo-Freudians such as Harry Stack Sullivan, Karen Horney, and Erich Fromm modified certain features of Freud's theory, and also played a major role in influencing conceptions about neurotic development. Sullivan, for example, stressed the interpersonal context of personality development and deemphasized the biologically oriented stages of psychosexual development.

The writings of Freud and the neo-Freudians served to further our understanding of neurotic development in several ways. First, they focused attention on early childhood development in the family context. Second, they emphasized the role of emotional-motivational factors and conflict. And in this context, they illustrated the functioning of the many avoidance strategies that people use in coping with negative affect and conflict. And third, Freud in particular opened our eyes to the existence of childhood sexuality and the role of sexuality generally in some adult disorders. Thus, the intensive study of individual cases that is the hallmark of Freudian and neo-Freudian therapy has produced a storehouse of ideas and theories that continue to influence our thinking about neurotic disorder.

Not all of the influence can be said to be positive. The main drawbacks to much of Freudian and neo-Freudian theory can be summarized as follows. First, these theories were based largely on the analysis of the memories, free associations, and dreams of middle- or upper-class *adults*. It is better if our theories derive directly from the phenomenon to be understood, in this case, the immediate (probably childhood) circumstances leading to the development of neurotic disorders.

Second, there is a tendency to take a few key concepts and apply them universally to all neurotic development. For example, traditional Freudian theory says that all neurotic disorders have their origins in an unsatisfactorily resolved oedipal conflict. While it may be true that an unresolved oedipal conflict played a primary role in the development of some neurotic disorders, it is highly unlikely that this is universally the case.

Third, the theories themselves are not stated systematically, and might best be described as a conglomeration of theories and propositions that are only loosely tied together. As a result, it is not meaningful to ask whether the theory as a whole is true or false, but only whether some one of the many theories is true. The general lack of coherence within these theories is made worse by a tendency for writers not to make a clear distinction between descriptive observations and theoretical inferences. They sometimes write as though an anal fixation or an oedipal conflict was directly observed when, in fact, what was observed was a verbal statement about "neatness" or an expression of anger at father. Also, in the course of theorizing there is a strong tendency to assume that a phenomenon has been explained if it is given a name. Thus, we "explain" a person's anxiety by saying that it is castration anxiety stemming from the oedipal conflict. Such explanations are almost always post-hoc in the sense that they are given after the fact and represent little more than attaching a label to an observed event, an anxiety reaction in this case. The theory has rarely been put to the test of predicting some reaction ahead of time. And finally, the theory is stated in such a fashion that most of it is probably not susceptible to disproof. That is, any particular empirical finding can be interpreted as being consistent with the theory.

In the remainder of this chapter and in the next chapter, we will examine evidence with respect to originating circumstances and current sustaining factors in the different varieties of neurotic disorders. Possible hereditary factors have already been reviewed, and the emphasis in these chapters will be on the role of learning experiences. In addition to reporting empirical evidence, which unfortunately remains skimpy, we will attempt to formulate testable hypotheses about neurosis development.

SOCIAL LEARNING IN THE FAMILY CONTEXT

For the young child the family is the most important context within which social learning occurs. We will, accordingly, focus on the family system, but this should not be taken to indicate that nonfamily experiences cannot be important. They can be, and we will take note of extra-familial circumstances from time to time.

Neurotic Parents

Statistical surveys have consistently shown that neurotic individuals tend to come from homes in which a higher proportion of parents have neurotic symptoms than in the general population (Jenkins, 1966; Shields, & Slater, 1961). Liverant (1959) found significantly more deviant Minnesota Multiphasic Personality Inventory profiles in parents of children referred to child guidance clinics than in parents of normal children. These empirical findings, of course, tell us nothing about the relative contribution of heredity and social learning; either, or more likely an interaction between the two, can readily account for the facts.

There is a tendency for married couples to be similar in terms of the presence or absence of neurotic disorder. Such a finding suggests that positive assortative mating has occurred, that is, neurotic individuals tend to marry other neurotic individuals and nonneurotics marry nonneurotics. Buck and Ladd, however, suggest that in addition to assortative mating there may be a tendency for similarity in neurotic status to increase with length of marriage. Such a finding suggests that either a neurotic spouse tends to produce neurotic reactions in a nonneurotic mate or a nonneurotic spouse helps a neurotic mate to overcome the neurotic reaction, or both. The evidence for progressive increase in similarity is not strong, however, and more research is necessary.

Neurotic disorder in one or both parents is likely to be accompanied by marital conflict. In recent years, the marriage relationship has been given central importance by many clinical writers as a focal point from which other neurosis-inducing social interactions derive (Satir, 1964). Cummings et al. (1966), for example, found that parents of emotionally disturbed or deviant children report more dissatisfaction and conflict with their spouse than do parents of normal children. Gassner and Murray (1969) found direct behavioral measures of interparent conflict to be higher in parents of neurotic than in parents of normal children. Ferreira and Winter (1968) found that in three-way (father-mother-child) interaction, families with a neurotic child exchanged less information, took longer to reach a decision and spent a greater proportion of time in silence.

Clinical reports suggest several likely ways in which disturbed marital interaction can form part of a larger system that includes children and can eventuate in child disturbance.

1. Simple displacement of anger and aggression from spouse to child may be the most common way. Say a wife is furious at her husband. Typical husband-wife interaction is such in this marriage that their anger is not expressed directly to each other, and underlying sources of frustration and disappointment are not confronted and dealt with. The wife may displace her anger to a child in the form of irrational temper outbursts inappropriate to the child's misbehavior, if any, or in chronic criticism and nagging.

2. Husband-wife antagonism, although originally stemming from other sources, may center around child rearing as one battlefield. For example, the husband accuses the wife of being too lax, or of being too hard on the girls but too easy on the boys. The wife says the husband does not pay any attention to disciplinary problems until things get out of hand and then he blows his stack. He leaves it to her but criticizes her for the way she handles it. Both the husband's and wife's reactions to the children become as much determined by their own conflict as by the reality of the child's behavior.

3. One spouse may attempt to enlist a child as an ally against the other spouse.

4. One spouse may react to the other with helplessness and withdrawal, and attempt to get a child to assume adult responsibility.

The possibilities are infinite. There is no reason, however, to suggest that *all* neurotic disorders develop in families with disturbed marital interaction or that disturbed marital interaction *always* results in neurotic disturbances in children. It is quite likely that in some instances rather serious marital discord is kept confined to the husband-wife dyad and not allowed to seriously affect parent-child interactions. Some degree of insight into the nature of displacement mechanisms would probably aid in keeping the marital conflict "encapsulated." It is also likely that there are numerous instances of disturbed parent-child interactions occurring in families where there is little or no marital conflict.

Anger and Aggression in Neurotic Disorder

Aggression is defined as behavior whose goal is the destruction or injury of some object or person. The emotion of anger is a likely, but not necessary, accompaniment of aggressive behavior. Both anger and associated aggressive tendencies are frequently involved in neurotic disorders. If a behavior disorder takes the form of purely aggressive "acting out" or antisocial behavior we are likely to apply a label such as delinquency, psychopathy, or antisocial reaction, but not consider it to be neurotic. On the other hand, childhood disorders involving a mixture of aggressive reactions and more characteristic neurotic symptoms such as phobic fears, poor peer relations, sleep disturbances, enuresis, crying spells, and facial mannerisms are quite common. For example, see Thomas et al. (1968). Also, clinical experiences with adult neurotics indicates the frequent presence of strong anger and aggressive urges that are inhibited and not ordinarily acted upon. Recall the murderous anger of the obsessive-compulsive woman described in Chapter 2.

Hyperactivity and aggressiveness in children can be associated with certain kinds of organic brain pathology caused, for example, by birth injury or encephalitis. We will not consider this type of causative factor except to say that an organically based disposition to aggressiveness can be magnified by the factors outlined below. The empirical results in the area of parent-child interaction as well as experimental studies with human and animal subjects suggest that three factors contribute to the strength of an aggressive response tendency in a particular situation.

1. The arbitrary interruption of goal-directed behavior, commonly called frustration, tends to produce an aggressive response, accompanied by the emotion of anger. It is not clear to what extent anger-aggression is an innate reaction to frustrations. Certainly the high-intensity emotional reaction that occurs in the young infant when his bottle is removed appears to have qualities of anger-aggression. Learning, of course, can also play a role in producing an association between frustrating circumstances and subsequent anger-aggression. An aggressive response to frustration may well be reinforced if it removes an interfering barrier or reinstitutes a withheld source of reinforcement. For example, someone is likely to return a displaced bottle to the mouth of a thrashing, yelling infant and thereby reinforce the aggressive response. Whether innate to some extent or not, the occasion of arbitrary frustration seems to serve commonly as a discriminative stimulus for anger-aggression in the human child.

Research has shown that parents of aggressive children are more likely to use arbitrary, power assertive, punitive disciplinary actions than parents of less aggressive children (Bandura & Walters, 1959; Baumrind, 1967; Kagan & Moss, 1962; McCord, McCord, & Howard, 1961; Shaefer & Bayley, 1963). In these studies the children were not institutionalized or being seen in clinics. Studies of parents of more extremely aggressive, antisocial children seen in clinics or institutions for delinquents yield similar findings (Glueck & Glueck, 1950; Lewis, 1954; Rosenthal et al., 1959; Rosenthal et al., 1962; Jenkins, 1968). Results in these latter studies are based primarily on parent interview or social worker case notes, but in contrast to the parent interview results for "normal," noninstitutionalized children there is a good deal of consistency in the findings. This empirical relationship may be explained in part if we assume that punitive parental actions frequently involve a frustration of the child's goal-directed behavior. Repeated frustrations of this kind would constantly instigate aggressive responses in the child.

2. The observation of another family member behaving in an aggressive way increases the probability that the child will also behave aggressively in similar situations. If aggressive behavior in another person is observed to achieve desired goals, then this should contribute further to the imitative tendency. The parent who uses punitive discipline accompanied by verbal and/or physical aggressiveness is providing a model for the child whether the aggression is directed toward the child or a sibling. Outside of controlled experimentation there is no way of knowing to what extent parent aggression toward the child is promoting aggressive child behavior by frustration or by modeling factors. Observed parental aggression toward a spouse or a neighbor would also provide additional modeling of aggression. McCord et al. (1961) report higher levels of overt conflict between parents of aggressive than parents of less aggressive boys.

Hetherington and Frankie (1967) studied the extent to which 4- to 6-year-old children imitated their father or mother. From a large pool of 310 families on which measures of parent dominance, interparent conflict and parent warmth–hostility had been obtained by direct observation in a standardized behavioral test situation, groups of 80 families with a male child and 80 with a female child were selected. Half of these children were from high-conflict homes and half from low-conflict homes. Within each conflict group half the subjects were from mother-dominant and half from father-dominant homes. Groups were further subdivided so that within each conflict-dominance group there were four warmth combinations: mother high–father low, mother low–father high, mother high–father high, and mother low–father low. Each child observed both parents on separate occasions make incidental postural, motor, and verbal responses associated with playing with a group of toys or games; for example, a parent might select a green toy and say, "green is my lucky color." The child was then permitted to play with the same materials.

Under mother dominance both boys and girls were more inclined to imitate incidental behavior in mother. Under father dominance boys imitated the father more while girls continued to imitate the mother more. The authors suggest that for boys in this age range a dominant father is especially facilitative of a shift from imitating the more feminine attributes of mother to the more masculine attributes of father. There was also a general tendency to imitate parents high on warmth more than parents who were hostile or punitive. Mussen and Parker (1965) also found that girls imitated nurturant mothers more than nonnurturant mothers.

In homes where parental conflict was high Hetherington and Frankie found more imitation of the dominant parent than in homes having low conflict. Perhaps under conditions of overt interparent conflict the behaviors associated with parent dominance are especially salient and thus more readily imitated by the child. This facilitation of dominant parent imitation under conditions of high interparent conflict was greater in mother-dominant than father-dominant homes. A finding of some interest relates to the conditions under which children will imitate a hostile, unfriendly parent, a response that goes contrary to the general tendency to imitate parents high on warmth. When both parents were rated low on warmth (relatively high on hostility and punitiveness) and high in interparent conflict, both boys and girls showed a strong tendency to imitate the dominant and, in this case, hostile parent. This finding suggests that when a child is confronted with two punitive parents in an atmosphere of interparent conflict he will imitate the more dominant (powerful!) parent in self-defense, that is, in order to placate or stay on the good side of this powerful and punitive figure. Imitation of this kind would be analogous to "identification with the aggressor" in psychoanalytic theory. However, when the nondominant parent was high on warmth, the tendency to imitate the dominant but hostile parent was markedly reduced. In this case the availability of a warm or accepting parent may provide a source of support for the child and reduce his need to placate the hostile parent.

3. Positive reinforcement following an aggressive response increases the strength of the response, and aversive consequences decrease the strength of the response. A child wants a piece of candy. The parent says no. The child throws a temper tantrum. The parent yields and gives the child the candy. The parent has reinforced the aggressive temper tantrum and increased the likelihood that it will be repeated on future occasions. Child aggression may be reinforced in many ways: for example, by obtaining some desired object from a peer, by finally getting an otherwise indifferent parent's attention, and by obtaining recognition and status from peers. Parents may reinforce certain kinds of child aggression with verbal approval; for example, children may be praised for sticking up for their rights and for various kinds of assertive behavior that blend into aggression. More rarely, some parents may subtly approve of child aggression because it gives them vicarious satisfaction for their own inhibited aggressive impulses. The approval in this case is not likely to be explicit, but rather communicated by the parents' intense interest in hearing about the behavior.

Patterson, Littman, and Bricker (1967) report findings that dramatically illustrate the influence of peer reinforcement in shaping aggressive behavior. When aggressive behavior by a nursery school child was followed by positive reinforcement (e.g., the other child gave up a toy or otherwise yielded), on one occasion it was found that the next time this child made an aggressive response it would tend to consist of the same type of aggression directed at the same victim. If on the first occasion the aggressive response had been followed by an aversive consequence (e.g., counterattack), the child would be more likely to change either the nature of the aggressive response or the victim the next time he made an aggressive response. Some children who had initially shown low rates of aggressive behavior increased dramatically in rate of aggressive behavior. Such large increases were associated with children who were frequently victimized by other children, but who at some point initiated a series of successful, and therefore reinforcing, counterattacks.

The proposition that aversive consequences following aggressive behavior decrease its strength is true in general, but there are some qualifications. When the aversive consequences take the form of punishment, the frustration and modeling features tend to increase aggressive response strength at the same time that the aversive consequences tend to cause a decrease. The results obviously can be complicated insofar as predicting the net increase or decrease in aggressive response. In this situation the aversive consequences should reduce aggression directed toward the punitive parent, but might result in an increase in displaced aggression toward siblings, peers, inanimate objects or pets.

When an aggressive response is followed by an aversive consequence that does not serve as a model for aggression, the strength of the aggressive response should decrease. Examples would be taking away a privilege or sending the child to his room without accompanying verbal scolding or physical punishment. A procedure that seems especially effective as an aversive consequence is the "Time Out" procedure whereby the child is put in a lighted and comfortable but relatively bare room for a period of about five minutes. If he continues to show aggressive, tantrum-type behavior additional five minute periods are added, so that his eventual release is associated with *not* being aggressive.

Parent inconsistency in punishing child aggression should correlate with high child aggression. The inconsistent parent may be one who is usually lax and permits aggression to pay off but occasionally reacts with irrational punitiveness and thus frustrates the child and models aggression. Another type of inconsistency would involve one parent who always punishes aggression and another parent who rarely, if ever, punishes aggression. In either case aggression is paying off for the child on a partial reinforcement schedule. Baumrind (1967) and McCord et al. (1961) found both kinds of inconsistency in parents of aggressive boys. Inconsistency should not be seen as involving any new factors—just a particular combination of the three basic ones.

As the language and conceptual skills of the child develop, the use of immediate consequences can be supplemented by verbal instruction. The parents can explain what the consequences of certain actions will be and the child can learn to "tell himself" symbolically about these consequences when his parents are not present. These thought processes can serve as discriminative stimuli that elicit controls on aggressive behavior. Self instructions of this kind play an important role not just in controlling aggressive behavior but in self-regulatory behavior generally as will be discussed in the next section of this chapter. If there is inconsistency between the verbal instructions from parents or from the child to himself and the actual consequences, there is likely to be less inhibition of aggression. In the case of such inconsistency, the actual consequences, positive or negative, will probably be much more influential than incorrect verbal statements about expected consequences.

We must not lose sight of the "systems" approach to personality development. There is a general tendency to emphasize parent causality in discussing the above factors, and it is reasonable to assume that parents *are* more influential in the system in the early years. Nevertheless early childhood traits, possibly influenced by heredity, such as hyperactivity or fussiness, may elicit parent reactions of greater punitiveness or criticalness than would otherwise have occurred. Once a system, parent punitiveness—child aggression for example, has developed, the question of cause and effect is no longer very meaningful. An aggressive child usually elicits more parent punitiveness and occasional "giving in" to coercive demands than a quiet, conforming child. Parent correlates such as general aggressiveness in other relationships and interparent conflict, however, are more likely to have been present before child aggressiveness developed and represent sources of parent influence *relatively* less affected by child reaction.

We will return to the role of anger-aggression in neurotic disorder but first we shall consider the development of self-regulatory behavior.

Self-regulation

Broadly speaking, the socialization process is concerned with "teaching" the child to behave in ways prescribed by society. This involves learning to stop doing certain things such as urinating and defecating in places other than the bathroom, crying or making other reactions inappropriate to a given age level, as well as learning new responses such as table manners, cooperative behavior, and educational achievement. It is unlikely that much early socialization learning can occur without external sources of reinforcement. That is, genetic dispositions or other internal states of the infant are not likely to produce even rudimentary aspects of socialized behavior without learning experiences provided by external sources of reinforcement. However, as the child grows older he does seem to develop the capacity to maintain already learned features of socially approved behavior under circumstances *where there is no obvious external reinforcement for this behavior*. There is no sharp demarcation between the presence or absence of external reinforcement in real life, but there are instances in which children (or adults) resist performing some tempting but disapproved act or atone for some past misdeed when it should be quite clear to the child that reinforcement, punishment in this case, is highly unlikely. Likewise children, or adults, will sometimes confess past misdeeds or seek out punishment when there is little likelihood of anyone ever finding out about the misdeed.

The term conscience has been commonly used to refer to self-regulatory behavior of this kind, and within psychoanalytic theory the term superego is used. Since there is a temptation to explain the behavior by saying it is the result of conscience or superego, we will stick to the more descriptive term, self-regulation, to refer to the behavior in question. One problem with research in this area is that different kinds of child behavior presumed to be indicative of self-regulation do not correlate highly, if at all, with each other. As mentioned in Chapter 5, Hartshorne and May (1928) found that children showed little consistency in cheating, lying, and stealing in different situations. More recently Sears, Rau, and Alpert (1965) found that behavioral measures of resistance to temptation obtained from four-year-old nursery school children did not correlate with measures of either tendency to confess or emotional upset after succumbing to temptation. Four different measures of resistance to temptation did, however, intercorrelate moderately well with a median correlation of .35 for boys and .44 for girls. Playing or not playing with a highly desirable toy after having been left alone in a room with instructions not to play with the toy is an example of one type of resistance to temptation measure used.

It is possible that resistance to temptation, whether highly situational or not, can be accounted for entirely on the basis of strong aversive consequences applied externally in the past. Responses are learned that avoid this aversive consequence, and these avoidance responses generalize to situations where external consequences are unlikely. The timing of the aversive consequence is an important factor in producing resistance to transgression in this way. Aronfreed and Reber (1966), for example, found that children who were punished by verbal disapproval (No!—that's for older boys) just as they were beginning to reach for an attractive but forbidden toy showed more subsequent resistance to temptation when alone than children punished immediately *after* making the forbidden response. In similar studies Aronfreed (1966), Parke and Walters (1967), and Walters, Parke, and Cane (1965) have also found that early punishment is associated with greater subsequent self-regulatory behavior than punishment given after transgression.

It seems unlikely that all self-regulatory behavior can be explained on the basis of avoidance responses learned to external punishments, which then generalize to situations where external punishments are improbable. For one thing a child should eventually learn to discriminate situations where he is likely to "get caught" from those where he is not likely to "get caught." If he refrains from committing the forbidden act only when he thinks the odds of getting caught are high, then he is not showing self-regulatory behavior as we define it. The problem is that in most life situations one cannot usually know with a high degree of certainty that external consequences for misbehavior will not occur. It may well be that we overrate the role of the "voice of conscience" in determining our "moral" behavior and that external sources of approval and disapproval are the more powerful factors. It is more flattering to think that the former rather than latter is true. Our beliefs along this line may well be themselves a product of the external approval we get for *saying* that we follow moral principles because of conscience rather than out of fear of getting caught for doing otherwise.

Nevertheless, there will probably turn out to be more to self-regulation than generalization of responses learned to external punishments. We would emphasize two additional factors: 1) mediating cognitions, and 2) affective reactions that become associated with anticipatory actions or thoughts related to transgression.

Mediating cognitions in the form of verbal self-instructions that clearly describe the approved and disapproved behaviors, and that clearly describe the positive and negative consequences associated with these respective behaviors can serve as controlling stimuli for appropriate behavior. Any features of parental "teaching" that would enhance the learning of these cognitions, such as clear verbal presentations of the rules and consequences, or requests that the child repeat or rehearse the rules, should further strengthen self-regulatory tendencies. Scolding or yelling that makes the teaching experience aversive would probably detract from the effectiveness of this kind of cognitive learning.

Sears et al. (1965) found that the mother's pressure for independence, responsiveness to the child, and use of reasoning (all measured from direct observation of mother-child interaction) correlated significantly with resistance to temptation in girls. These results are consistent with the proposition that the mother of a self-regulating child is highly active in verbally describing desired behavior and providing reasons for it.

Experimental studies with young children further substantiate the effectiveness of verbal instructions, or cognitive structuring, in promoting resistance to temptation (Aronfreed, 1966; Liebert, Hanratty, & Hill, 1969; O'Leary, 1967; Parke, 1969). Parke, for example, found that verbal instructions in the form of giving the child a reason for not playing with a certain toy, "I don't want the toys to get broken or worn out. No one could use them anymore," increased resistance to temptation in first and second grade boys. Furthermore, the timing (early or somewhat delayed) or intensity of punishment (loudness or an unpleasant buzzer) or nurturance of the experimenter were less influential under high cognitive structure, suggesting that cognitive structuring was the more powerful variable.

Research has also been done on the question of whether verbal self-instructions taught or modeled by a nurturant person are more effective than those taught by a nonnurturant person. Results are equivocal. Nurturance is usually manipulated by having the child play with or observe a friendly, highly rewarding experimenter or model prior to the other procedures. Both social (smiling, talking, helping) and material (toys, candy) rewards may be given noncontingently to the child.

Parke (1969), as mentioned previously, found that children showed more resistance to temptation with a nurturant than a nonnurturant experimenter under conditions of low cognitive structure, but that under conditions of high cognitive structure the degree of nurturance of the experimenter did not have a significant effect.

Rosenhan and White (1967), however, found no effect of a prior friendly versus a prior critical experience with a model in 4th- and 5th-graders' imitation of altruistic behavior, giving away valued gift certificates to needy orphans. Bandura, Grusec, and Menlove (1967) found that high nurturance in a model actually decreased the tendency of the child to imitate high performance standards for self-reward relative to a low nurturant model. The latter results suggest that noncontingent nurturance is conducive of self-indulgence in the form of rewarding oneself for substandard performance.

Thus the effect of parent nurturance on self-regulation remains unclear. If the response involves incidental and stylistic aspects of behavior then a noncontingently nurturant parent may enhance imitation as found in the previously described studies of Hetherington and Frankie (1967) and Mussen and Parker (1965). If the response involves resistance to temptation and restraint then noncontingent nurturance in the parent may have only weak effects or perhaps actually lower self-regulatory tendencies.

The second factor involves the association of affect responses to anticipatory actions or mediating cognitions. A common interpretation of the effectiveness of early as opposed to late punishment is that some negative affect, such as anxiety, becomes associated with anticipatory actions or thoughts related to transgression. The child reduces the negative affect by inhibiting the forbidden response. Parents are likely to be inducing affective reactions in the child when the child is learning verbal instructions about approved and disapproved behavior and their respective consequences. The prior learning of empathic emotional responses, as discussed in Chapter 5 should greatly facilitate the association of affective reactions to occasions of parental approval and disapproval. By empathic emotional response we mean responding to the observation of the overt manifestations of another person's emotional response with a similar emotional response. It is easy to imagine how such empathic responses might be learned by the young child. A mother, for example, who is unhappy, irritable, frightened, or otherwise distressed is likely to behave toward the child in ways that produce a negative emotional reaction in the child. On the other hand a mother who is happy, smiling and contented is more likely to facilitate a similar positive emotional reaction in the child. After repeated pairings of this sort, the overt manifestations of mother's emotional reaction, her facial expression, tone of voice, etc., can come to elicit similar, empathic emotions in the child. As the child develops, mediating cognitions of the kind, "he was struck by a rock and that hurts; his mother got mad and yelled at him," can come to elicit empathic emotional responses. As a result direct observation of the other person's expressive behavior is no longer necessary for the occurrence of empathic emotional responses. And in time it may not be necessary to directly observe the events at all. A person can simply be told, or tell himself, that such and such happened to so and so, and experience an empathic emotional reaction.

The role of empathic responses in the learning of altruistic behavior was demonstrated in a study by Aronfreed and Paskal (1968). Positive affective reactions in 6- to 8-year-old children were first attached to expressive cues in an adult that were meant to reflect a corresponding positive or pleasurable affective state. The adult sat next to the child and demonstrated the operation of two levers. Pushing one lever produced a small piece of candy and pushing the other lever resulted in a red light being on for three seconds. Each outcome occurred only 60 percent of the time. The adult showed no reaction when candy was dispensed or when nothing happened. But when the red light went on, the adult expressed positive affect by smiling while staring at the light, and exclaiming in a pleased and excited tone of voice, "There's the light!" The adult then hugged the child with one arm, and smiled broadly at the child.

The children were then allowed to operate the levers on their own. Children who had been given the prior opportunity to learn an empathic response were subsequently more willing to forego candy in order to push the lever that would result in the adult showing the expressive cues associated with pleasure than were children in several control conditions. In another study Aronfreed and Paskal (1968) taught children to respond to overt expressions of distress in an adult with empathic distress of their own, and demonstrated that this prior learning was an important factor in the subsequent manifestation of sympathetic behavior—actions aimed at relieving another child's distress.

The development of self-regulatory behavior, then, may be greatly facilitated by the prior learning of strong empathic responses. Given this prior learning, a parent who by tone of voice and facial expression, as well as by verbal content, is showing emotional distress would be producing an empathic negative affect response in the child in addition to any other distress produced by specific, external punishments. Future occasions of temptation should not only elicit the mediating cognitions (I should not do that. Mother will be mad at me. I may get punished.) but also some negative affect associated with anticipatory transgression and perhaps positive affect associated with resisting temptation. Under these circumstances a child may develop a powerful mechanism of *self-reinforcement* to use in the regulation of his own behavior.

When conditions are such as to produce unusually strong negative affect associated with thoughts of parent disapproval, neurotically inhibiting degrees of self-regulation may occur that generalize beyond the family situation. This might be particularly facilitated when the child has few sources of external reinforcement, and has to rely heavily on self-reinforcements obtained by thoughts and fantasy. Within the framework of psychoanalytic theory many neurotics are characterized as having an overly strict superego.

Other features of self-regulatory behavior involving tendencies to confess or to seek punishment may result in part from straightforward reinforcement for doing these things. Some parents praise, forgive, or otherwise reinforce the child when he confesses. Parent forgiveness after punishment may be a powerful reinforcer for punishment seeking behavior for the child who has come to experience parental disapproval as strongly aversive. Because confessing and seeking punishment received strong reinforcement in the past the responses may be repeated in the future even though there is little likelihood that the parents would otherwise have found out about the misbehavior. Perhaps confessing and seeking punishment should not be considered as self-regulatory since there is little evidence to suggest that they are positively correlated with behavioral resistance to temptation.

Baumrind (1967) conducted a study that supports many of the proposals about the development of both aggression and self-regulatory responses. This study also incorporated many desirable methodological features, and is worth describing in some detail. Three groups of children were selected from a larger group of 110 3- to 4-year-old nursery school children (male and female) on the basis of 14 weeks of behavioral observation. The 13 children in group I (energetic-friendly) were rated higher on each of the following than either of the other two groups: self-reliance, approach to novel or stressful situations with interest and curiosity, self-control, energy level, cheerful mood, and friendly peer relations. The differences between the 11 children in group II (conflicted-irritable) and the 8 children in group III (impulsive-aggressive) children might be summarized as follows: Group II children showed more self-control and self-reliance than Group III but less than Group I. Group II children were inclined to be less cheerful and recover from expressions of annoyance more slowly than Group III. In general Group II would seem to involve a more conflicted group of children in which aggressions and unfriendly reactions alternate with more socially withdrawn behavior: and unhappy, irritable, and apprehensive mood states prevail. These children may represent a high risk group with respect to future neurotic development. Group III children seem to be more purely impulsive and lacking in self-discipline of any kind.

Parent behavior was assessed in three ways: (a) in the homes, (b) in a structured observation procedure (mother only), and (c) by interview. The observational procedures permitted the functional analysis of certain interactional patterns. Interaction sequences were identified which were initiated by either the parent or child and involved some demand upon the other person. The various responses were then coded in terms of the way in which the person attempted to gain compliance (for example, a parent might offer positive incentives or use arbitrary power) and whether or not the other person complied. It was determined whether the parent did or did not persist in his demand after an initial noncompliance from the child, or the extent to which the parent succumbed to the child's "nuisance value," that is, was coerced into complying by the child's whining, pleading or crying.

The structured observation procedure involved two parts: a) the mother teaching the child some simple mathematical concepts and b) a free play period. This interaction was coded in a number of ways, including compliance or noncompliance to demands as described above.

Results indicated a strong tendency for parents of Group I children (energetic-friendly) relative to both other groups to exert more control over their children and be less affected by coercive demands based on whining and crying. This kind of control is not necessarily punitive, unduly restrictive, or intrusive. It would seem to reflect the parent's ability to resist pressure from the child and the parent's willingness to exert influence upon the child.

Parents of Group I children also made more maturity demands where information and reasons were given for the demands. They also more often explicitly retracted a demand on the basis of the child's arguments. The latter is different from succumbing to the child's nuisance value in that the parent explicitly indicates that the demand is being modified on the basis of a specific argument advanced by the child. In other words, parents of Group I children permitted and to some extent encouraged independent thought and action but did not allow themselves to be coerced by noxious child behavior. Parents of Group I children were also more nurturant as indicated by a greater percentage of child-initiated sequences which resulted in satisfaction for the child, including those involving the child's request for support and attention. Greater nurturance was also indicated by the tendency for Group I parents to use more positive reinforcement and less punishment than other parents.

In summary, Group I parents, relative to both Group II and III parents, provided high nurturance with high control, high demands with clear communication about what was required, and a willingness to listen and occasionally be influenced by the child's point of view. These results are portrayed in Figure 10 where measures are combined to form four general

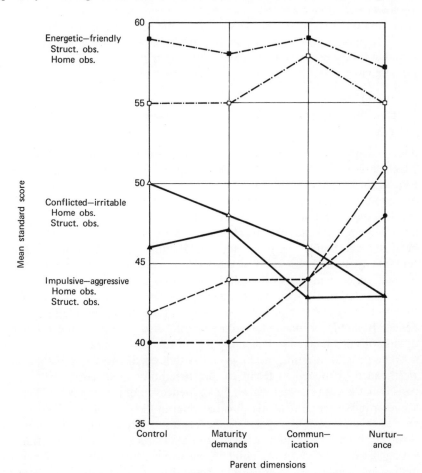

FIGURE 10. Profile of composited parent dimension scores from the summary rating for the structured observation and the home visit sequence analysis for each group (Adapted from Baumrind, 1967).

categories: control, maturity demands, clear communication, and nurturance.

Groups II (conflicted-irritable) and III (impulsive-aggressive) differed from each other in that parents of Group III were less persistent in the face of child opposition to enforce demands, and succumbed more to child nuisance value. Group III parents also provided less maturity demands, and tended to be more nurturant (difference not statistically significant) than Group II parents. A father interview measure indicated greater use of corporal punishment by Group II than Group III fathers, further suggesting lower nurturance as well as greater punitiveness in Group II. The children in Group II would seem to show neuroticlike conflict over the expression of aggression, which would be consistent with the combination of aggression producing and aggression inhibiting factors present in the parent behavior.

Negative Affect, Conflict, and Avoidance Strategies

Although there are many clinical reports about possible neurosis-inducing aspects of family interaction, there are practically no studies in which groups of families with a child manifesting a specific kind of neurotic disorder have been compared with nonneurotic control families on behaviorally oriented measures of relevant family interaction. Ideally the child would be young and the neurotic process would still be in a developmental phase. The studies of Thomas et al. (1968) on the interaction of heredity and family learning, and the Baumrind (1967) study just described represent good starts in the right direction. Much of what follows in this section must unfortunately be based on studies of individual families, and should be seen as an attempt to formulate testable hypotheses rather than as a statement of conclusions based on strong empirical evidence. It should be understood that reference to parents in the following discussion can be taken to mean any significant other person.

The general question can be posed as follows. If two groups of families were exactly matched in terms of any hereditary predispositions to neurosis, what kinds of social learning experiences in one group would lead to a higher incidence of neurotic disorder than in the other group? We would answer this question by suggesting that the following factors are commonly involved in the development of neurotic disorders: 1) the induction of strong negative affect in the child, 2) the creation of conflict involving simultaneous tendencies to approach or avoid interaction with parents, or to express or inhibit responses associated with reactions such as anger-aggression, grief, sex, etc., 3) the learning of avoidance strategies that minimize the negative affect.

Illustrative cases. Some examples may serve to clarify these factors. Donald R., Jr., age 10, and his father and mother were seen in brief family therapy (six sessions in two weeks) as part of a small pilot study (Martin, 1967). He was described by his teacher on a behavioral check list as being subject to crying spells, explosive outbursts of temper, not having any friends, constantly seeking help and reassurance from the teacher, and failing in his course work. He had already been held back one year because of poor academic performance. The family background was upper middle class and his intelligence test performance was considerably above average.

Mr. R. had by his own report been given to irrational outbursts of anger and criticism toward Donald since an early age and was also inclined to give lectures to Donald on the importance of being responsible, and living up to his name which had apparently been handed down from several generations of successful Donald R.'s. In one session the father, at the request of the therapist, had told Donald how angry he felt when Donald disobeyed, including wishing at times that Donald had never been born. The impact of this expression on Donald was marked. He began to tremble and cry, and, when asked to tell his father about his reaction, described a painful tightness in his stomach and how scared he was of his father's anger. The negative affect arousal, whatever emotional label might be attached to it, was obviously an extremely unpleasant experience. Although Donald was able to express some anger at his father (well justified anger in view of the father's irrational attacks) in the course of the sessions, his most prominent type of expression involved statements that paraphrased his father's lectures—how he should be responsible, study hard, obey the household rules, do his chores and generally bring honor to the family name. Such a reaction might be conceived as "identification with the aggressor" in psychoanalytic theory, but it would seem most readily explainable as an attempt to placate his father, that is to turn off his aversive outbursts by saying the right things. Unfortunately the father's irrational attacks were not highly contingent on clear-cut instances of misbehavior, and were inappropriately intense in any case. Donald's attempts to verbally placate his father were probably reinforced to some extent by his father's getting "off his back" but were far from successful in preventing attacks. By the time the family was seen Donald was indeed performing at an ineffective level in many areas and was thus providing his father with more than enough excuses for attacking him.

This example illustrates the three factors previously listed. The induction of strong negative affect is clearly present. Conflict seems to center around any kind of approach, physical or verbal, to the father. The expression of anger-aggression to the father is almost completely inhibited and overt aggression is displaced to siblings, peers, or teachers. The primary avoidance strategy shown is the tendency to placate his father by verbally repeating his father's lectures. The fact that his father's aversive responses were not contingent on some criterion of reasonable performance by Donald may have special relevance for the development of neurotic disorder. If his father's aversive responses were more contingent, Donald would probably have learned to perform in ways that would prevent his father's punishing reactions, and this continuing source of negative affect would not be present. Highly contingent punishments applied in many areas might, on the other hand, have led to over conformity and inhibition. As it is, Donald rather desperately but unsuccessfully tries to prevent his father's irrational attacks by verbal promises about behaving properly. Donald has not learned an effective avoidance strategy at this time, and the neurotic disorder consists primarily of expressions of the negative affect.

Consider another example. Jerry B., age 10, was seen with his father and mother as part of a study on family interaction correlates of child aggression, withdrawal, and nondeviancy (Martin and Hetherington, 1971). Jerry was rated as highly withdrawn and fearful by both his teacher and his peers. As part of a standardized experimental procedure Jerry and his father were asked to talk to each other and reach agreement about a recurring conflict between them. Some verbatim excerpts from this interaction are shown below. In this interaction the father's voice is highly controlled and relatively emotionless. He never smiles or expresses humor. For Jerry it is clearly an unpleasant experience but he shows no strong display of emotion other than a rather tense posture. The topic under discussion involves Jerry's tendency to avoid practicing knot tying (for Boy Scouts) and the difficulty he has in tying knots under time pressure.

> FATHER: Well, what's . . . what seemed to be wrong, that you couldn't tie these knots?
> JERRY: Well, I got a little tongue-tied.
> FATHER: Tongue-tied. You don't tie your knots with your tongue, do you?
> JERRY: Hum.
> FATHER: Huh?
> JERRY: No.
> FATHER: Well?
> JERRY: I got confused.
> FATHER: He gets confused. Why didn't you seem to control yourself? You seemed to go out of control, didn't you?
> JERRY: Yeah.
> FATHER: Well, why do you think this happened?
> JERRY: I don't know.
> FATHER: You don't know.
> JERRY: No. Uh.
> FATHER: Well, if you don't, who does?

JERRY: I get all excited about tying them.
FATHER: Then you get overexcitement.
JERRY: Um-hum (yes).
FATHER: You think that overexcitement gets you flustered?
JERRY: Yeah.
FATHER: Well, what do you think you can do about it?
JERRY: Oh, count . . . count . . . take it back and count to ten.
FATHER: Do you think that's going to calm you down?
JERRY: Um.
FATHER: Hum?
JERRY: I hope so.
FATHER: You hope so. Well, then, do you think we can come to this agreement?
JERRY: Uh-huh (yes).
FATHER: Well, I think we've solved the problem.

It is not surprising that Jerry becomes upset and confused when tying knots, especially under the tutelage of his father, given the aversive criticism associated with the knot-tying experience. Note that the father of this inhibited-withdrawn boy is explicitly teaching him to control emotional expression by counting to ten, remaining calm, and so on.

At a later point in the session Jerry was asked to express *his* feelings and *his* point of view when in this situation. The father was told to say nothing, just listen. Jerry said the following:

Well, I feel pretty bad, and I should calm down. I should count . . . take a deep breath and count to ten. Like this. And then I'll feel much better. And I hope in the future I won't lose my head, and calm down and count to ten, and I wish that everybody doesn't get as upset. I shouldn't go all to pieces. I'll pull myself together. And I feel like I really ought to count to twenty. And if I'm really low, I should count to . . . take two deep breaths, count to twenty and take a drink.

Most of the response is devoted to parroting the father's rules for remaining calm—the same placating characteristic observed in Donald R. About the only exception is the wish "that everybody doesn't get as upset," an indication of how aversive it is for him when father and others criticize him in this way.

Sometimes a child such as Jerry becomes so dominated by the one motive, to placate a critical parent, that he overdoes it and his very placating responses become a stimulus for more criticism, as occurred in the following interaction. Jerry and his father are discussing Jerry's tendency to get flustered when he is setting up camp in the Boy Scouts.

FATHER: Well, I felt pretty low. I asked you to do something, and there was nobody, everybody seemed to look at you, and then I felt pretty cheap, cause you didn't do what I asked you. Now how'd you feel about it?

JERRY: Well, I felt the same. I felt pretty low.

FATHER: Is there anything else?

JERRY: Well, I felt angry.

FATHER: How angry?

JERRY: Well, not too angry, but a little.

FATHER: Is this all you felt?

JERRY: Well, I felt bad too, cause everybody was looking at me. I should have put down the stick and handed out all the stakes.

FATHER: You think you need to correct this from now on?

JERRY: Yes.

FATHER: You do what people ask you to . . .

JERRY: And I don't need to . . . I'll hand out . . . do the most important thing first. And then I'll . . .

FATHER: Do, well, do which important thing?

JERRY: Do the most important thing first.

FATHER: Which most important? Your most important thing or what . . .

JERRY: Everybody else's most important thing. [Desperately tries to figure out what father wants him to say.]

FATHER: Well, that isn't the right either, is it? [Goes too far for father, who criticizes him for that.]

JERRY: Um, well, see, this is . . . [Confused now, does not know what father wants.]

FATHER: Suppose some boy wants . . . wish you to do something. Is it fair for you to do this?

JERRY: No . . . well, well, if he's in dire need of help.

FATHER: Oh.

EXPERIMENTER: Any other feeling on this matter?

JERRY: No.

A characteristic of the family systems of both Donald R. and Jerry B. is a kind of vicious circle in which as a direct result of certain features of parent-child interaction the child begins to behave in certain new ways that elicit more parent criticism, which further aggravate the child's symptoms. Donald R. began to perform poorly in school and behave "irresponsibly" at home, and Jerry B. becomes flustered and cannot perform satisfactorily in many situations, including Boy Scout activities. A variation occurs when parents have reinforced and are initially satisfied with a certain kind of child behavior, for example, immature behavior in a 4-year-old or passivity or femininity in a young boy, and then later become critical of this behavior.

Emotion in the form of negative affect has clearly been given a central role in our formulation of neurotic disorders. It is therefore of some interest to note that individuals involved in neurotic interaction systems frequently deny the presence of these disturbing emotions. Using parent interview and questionnaire type data, Sarason et al. (1960) found that mothers of high-anxiety elementary school children (boys and girls) were more defensive than mothers of low-anxiety children in responding to interview questions about their children. Mothers of high-anxiety children were more likely to deny anxiety symptoms in the child and generally describe him (or her) in a positive way even though the children themselves on self-report anxiety scales admitted many anxieties, worries, and fears. The fathers of the anxious children were less defensive and their reports about the child were more in line with the children's reports. The mothers' denial of anxiety in the children suggests that these mothers would find aversive any attempt on the child's part to tell her about his anxiety or emotional distress. She might respond to any such attempt by "shaming" him, changing the subject, or with some other aversive or at least nonreinforcing consequence. The child would eventually learn to conceal these experiences from her, and perhaps from others as well.

Another example illustrates this feature as well as the presence of strong negative affect. Johnny Z. was rated by teachers and peers as being both aggressive and socially isolated from his peers—somewhat similar to Donald R. He is talking with his mother about coming home in a bad mood because of some academic frustration at school.

MOTHER: How would you like to change that from happening? About your coming in the door and slamming your books down, and slamming the door and all of these things? What do you think you'd like to do?

JOHNNY: Tear up the place.

MOTHER: Do you think that would solve your problem?

JOHNNY: No.

MOTHER: Well, how . . . how would it solve your problem? What's best for you to solve your problem?

JOHNNY: Do it over.

MOTHER: Do it over? Well, how about if you came home from school and even if you were upset like that, do you think if you just hung up your coat and went upstairs with your books and came back downstairs and told me about it . . . come into the kitchen and told me about it, without having this big entrance?

JOHNNY: No.

MOTHER: You don't think you should come in and tell me? Well, it's upset you and it's going to upset you until you talk about it. Isn't it?

JOHNNY: Yeah.

MOTHER: Don't you think coming in the kitchen and talking to me would help you? Without slamming your books and without bickering at the other kids and things like that? Or do you just think if you came home from school and went upstairs and changed your clothes and then came down and talked to me, that would, . . . by that time it wouldn't be so important anyway.

JOHNNY: Yeah.

The mother is generally trying to get him to go to his room and calm down and preferably not bother her at all with his troubles at school. The following excerpt is taken from later in the session when he is asked to express his emotions and his point of view and mother has been told to just listen.

> Feels like I'm going to burst open and feel like I want to tear the place to pieces, then another feeling I don't like is feeling like smashing something to pieces. Then burning up the place, tearing down anything in my way, that's about all.

The intensity of his anger is further indicated in another part of the session where he talked about wanting to tear his clothes in small pieces, burn them, and throw them in the garbage can. The primary affect is anger but phrases such as, "I feel like a disease strikes me; I'm going to burst open; I'm nervous and I'm shaked to pieces," suggested a more complex emotional reaction and one that is certainly an aversive experience for him. In the quoted example the negative affect is not specifically instigated by the parent, but presumably by a frustration at school. However, on the basis of structured interaction obtained with the father, it was clear that Johnny experienced considerable aversive criticism from him, which may have been another source of anger instigation.

Anger and aggression in neurotic conflict. These examples further illustrate the central role of anger and aggression in the development of *some* neurotic disorders. Theoretical speculations about the development of neurotic conflict centering around anger-aggression might be summarized as follows. As found by Baumrind (1967) conflict is expected to develop when parents combine the instigation of anger-aggression in a nonnurturant context with moderate degrees of control and cognitive structuring designed to inhibit the expression of anger-aggression. It is likely that in the process of inhibiting direct expressions of anger-aggression parents would induce other affective reactions such as fear, grief, or shame. Thus, the child could begin to show complex affective reactions involving mixtures of, or rapid alternations between, anger, fear, grief, and shame—the picture of the irritable, moody child.

In subsequent development different kinds of avoidance strategies could be learned, largely on the basis of the particular models observed and reinforcement contingencies experienced: not thinking about aggression-arousing thoughts; intellectualization that results in detached, unemotional, and therefore nonangry states; cognitive interpretations, denials, or rationalizations that change the meaning of a situation so that aggression is not appropriate; and behavior traits of nonaggressiveness, passivity, submissiveness, courteousness, or formality that are incompatible with aggressiveness and also are less likely to elicit aggressive responses in others.

Varying degrees of stimulus displacement could occur (to siblings, pets, peers, teachers, employers, and inanimate objects) depending upon the degree of aversiveness associated with aggression toward parents or other original targets of aggression, similarity of the displacement object to the original target, and the type of reinforcement obtained for the displaced response. Varying degrees of response displacement could occur that depend upon the same factors. For example, responses might be displaced from physical assault or shouted insults to low intensity grumbling or sullen pouting.

Sex and other behavioral systems in neurotic conflict. Conflicts and defense mechanisms surrounding anxiety-arousing sexual impulses form the foundations of the psychoanalytic theory of neurosis (Fenichel, 1945). It is unlikely that sexual conflict plays a primary causative role in *all* neurotic disorders. On the other hand, it is true that disturbances in sexual functioning are a common concomitant of many neurotic disorders and conflict over sexual expression does play a central role in *some* cases.

The prevalence of sexual disturbance in neurotic disorders probably occurs for two reasons. 1) Sexual arousal and functioning is very much affected by emotional reactions such as fear, grief, shame, and also by the state of fatigue. And strong emotions and states of fatigue are common in neurotic disorders. 2) Since disturbed interpersonal relationships are a common feature of neurosis it is not surprising that inhibitions and conflicts present in other areas of interaction would also be reflected in that most intimate of relationships—sexual intercourse.

Sexuality becomes involved in neurotic disorder in a more primary way because it is a highly learnable response, readily conditioned to all kinds of stimuli, and also because conflict is frequently produced as a result of parents or others inducing negative affect in association with sexual expression. Thus, the highly learnable sexual response can become associated with members of the same sex (homosexuality), fetishistic objects such as articles of clothing, or behaviors such as stealing or setting fires. Sexual responses can also become associated with anger-aggression as seen in certain sadistic tendencies or with pain, humiliation, or other forms of punishment inflicted on oneself as seen in certain masochistic tendencies. In all of the above it is likely that there were childhood associations, perhaps on a chance basis, between strong sexual arousal and the behavior or emotion in question; for example, between sexual arousal and an angry-aggressive expression or an occasion of painful punishment. The subsequent compulsive nature of the behavior is readily accounted for on the basis of the strong, immediate positive affect (sexual arousal and possibly orgasm) outweighing more delayed aversive consequences of the act. The behavior may also continue in a compulsive way because the positive affect of sexual arousal is being used to reduce sources of negative affect that have no relation at all to sexuality in the same way that the alcoholic or the obese individual reduces life's aversiveness by drinking or eating, respectively.

When a strong approach-avoidance conflict exists with respect to sexual expression and inhibition one can find the same complex kinds of displacements and other avoidance strategies as were previously described for conflicts centering around aggression. For example, a college girl experienced occasions of unusual visual acuity in which everything was seen with exquisite sharpness, whereas ordinarily her vision appeared to be so poor as to require glasses. The periods of unusual visual acuity were accompanied by an unexplained mixture of excitement and apprehension, and one example she gave of the experience occurred while she was in a classroom looking at a handsome instructor. In a few psychotherapy sessions it was possible to identify the excitement as sexual arousal. In this case, visual functioning, the act of looking, had become "sexualized" by which we mean only that a strong association had developed, and the girl had learned by some kind of muscular control to see poorly as a way of avoiding negative affect that for her was associated with sexual interest. The avoidance response was relaxed occasionally and the sexualized looking with unusual visual acuity occurred (in contrast to her usual poor acuity).

Any motive or behavioral system can become part of the neurotic conflict: aggression; sex; achievement in academic, business, athletic, or social areas; interpersonal friendliness or intimacy; etc. The specific description of the behavior system involved is important in understanding and treating a given case. No attempt will be made to provide a catalog of examples of neurotic disorder as they might involve these various aspects of behavior. The general principles being developed should apply to most specific occurrences.

REFERENCES

Aronfreed, J. The internalization of social control through punishment: Experimental studies of the role of conditioning and the second signal system in the development of conscience. *Proceed. Eighteenth Internat. Congr. Psychol.,* Moscow, 1966.

Aronfreed, J., & Pascal, V. Altruism, empathy, and the conditioning of positive affect. Unpublished study described in Aronfreed, J. *Conduct and Conscience.* New York: Academic Press, 1968, 143–146.

Aronfreed, J., & Reber, A. Internalized behavioral suppression and the timing of social punishment. *J. pers. soc. Psychol.,* 1965, **1**, 3–16.

Bandura A., Gruesec, J. E., & Menlove, F. L. Some social determinants of self-monitoring reinforcement systems. *J. pers. soc. Psychol.,* 1967, **5**, 449–455.

Bandura, A., & Rosenthal, T. L. Vicarious classical conditioning as a function of arousal level. *J. pers. soc. Psychol.*, 1966, **3**, 54–62.

Bandura, A., & Walters, R. H. *Adolescent aggression*. New York: Ronald, 1959.

Baumrind, D. Child care practices anteceding three patterns of preschool behavior. *Genetic Psychol. Monogr.*, 1967, **75**, 43–88.

Berger, S. M. Conditioning through vicarious instigation. *Psychol. Rev.*, 1962, **69**, 450–466.

Buck, C. W., & Ladd, K. L. Psychoneurosis in marital partners. *Brit. J. Psychiat.*, 1965, **111**, 587–590.

Cummings, S. T., Bayley, H. C., & Rie, H. E. The effects of the child's deficiency on the mother: A study of mothers of mentally retarded, chronically ill and neurotic children. *Amer. J. Orthopsychiat.*, 1966, **36**, 595–608.

Fenichel, O. *The psychoanalytic theory of neurosis*. New York: Norton, 1945.

Ferreira, A. J., & Winter, W. D. Information exchange and silence in normal and abnormal families. *Family Process*, 1968, **7**, 251–276.

Gassner, S., & Murray, E. J. Dominance and conflict in the interactions between parents of normal and neurotic children. *J. abnorm. soc. Psychol.*, 1969, **74**, 33–41.

Glueck, S., & Glueck, E. T. *Unraveling Juvenile Delinquency*. Cambridge, Mass.: Harvard University Press, 1950.

Hetherington, E. M., & Frankie, G. Effects of parental dominance, warmth, and conflict on imitation in children. *J. pers. soc. Psychol.*, 1967, **6**, 119–125.

Jenkins, R. L. Psychiatric syndromes in children and their relation to family background. *Amer. J. Orthopsychiat.*, 1966, **36**, 450–457.

Jenkins, R. L. The varieties of children's behavioral problems and family dynamics. *Amer. J. Psychiat.*, 1968, **124**, 1440–1445.

Kagan, J., & Moss, H. A. *Birth to Maturity: A Study in Psychological Development*, New York: Wiley, 1962.

Lewis, H. *Deprived Children*. London: Oxford Univer. Press, 1954.

Liebert, R. M., Hanratty, M., & Hill, J. H. Effects of rule structure and training method on the adoption of a self-imposed standard. *Child Develop.*, 1969, **40**, 93–101.

Liverant, S. MMPI differences between parents of disturbed and nondisturbed children. *J. consult. Psychol.*, 1959, **23**, 256–260.

Martin, B. Family interaction associated with child disturbance: Assessment and modification. *Psychotherapy: Theory, Research and Practice*, 1967, **4**, 30–35.

Martin, B., & Hetherington, E. M. Family interaction correlates of child aggression, withdrawal and nondeviancy. In preparation.

McCord, W., McCord, J., & Howard, A. Familial correlates of aggression in nondelinquent male children. *J. abnorm. soc. Psychol.*, 1961, **62**, 79–83.

Mussen, P., & Parker, A. L. Mother nurturance and girls' incidental imitative learning. *J. pers. soc. Psychol.*, 1965, **2**, 94–97.

O'Leary, K. D. The effects of verbal and nonverbal training on learning and immoral behavior. Paper presented at Amer. Psychol. Assoc., Washington, D. C., 1967.

Parke, R. D. Effectiveness of punishment as an interaction of intensity, timing, agent nurturance and cognitive structuring. *Child Develop.*, 1969, **40**, 213–235.

Parke, R. D., & Walters, R. H. Some factors influencing the efficacy of punishment training for inducing response inhibition. *Monogr. soc. res. Child Develop.*, 1967, **32**, No. 1.

Patterson, G. R., Littman, R. A., & Bricker, W. Assertive behavior in children: a step towards a theory of aggression. *Monogr. soc. res. Child Develop.*, 1967.

Pond, D., Ryle, A., & Hamilton, M. Marriage and neurosis in a working-class population. *Brit. J. Psychiat.*, 1963, **109**, 592–598.

Rosenhan, D., & White, G. M. Observation and rehearsal as determinants of pro-social behavior. *J. pers. soc. Psychol.*, 1967, **5**, 424–431.

Rosenthal, M. J., Finkelstein, M., Ni, E., & Berkwits, G. K. A study of mother-child relationships in the emotional disorders of children. *Genetic Psychol. Monogr.*, 1959, **60**, 65–116.

Rosenthal, M. J., Ni, E., Finkelstein, M. & Berkwits, G. K. Father-child relationships and children's problems. *AMA Arch. gen. Psychiat.*, 1962, **7**, 360–373.

Sarason, S. B., Davidson, K. S., Lighthall, F. F., Waite, R. R., & Ruebush, B. K. *Anxiety in elementary school children.* New York: Wiley, 1960.

Satir, V. *Conjoint family therapy.* Palo Alto: Science and Behavior Books, 1964.

Sears, R. R., Rau, L., & Alpert, R. *Identification and Child Training.* Stanford, Calif.: Stanford University Press, 1965.

Shaefer, E. S., & Bayley, N. Maternal behavior, child behavior and their inter-correlations from infancy through adolescence. *Child Develop. Monogr.*, 1963, **281**, Whole No. 3.

Shields, J., & Slater, E. Heredity and Psychological abnormality. In H. J. Eysenck (Ed.), *Handbook of abnormal psychology.* New York: Basic Books, 1961.

Thomas, A., Chess, S., & Birch, H. G. *Temperament and behavior disorders in children.* New York: New York University Press, 1968.

Walters, R. H., Parke, R. D., & Cane, V. Timing of punishment and the observation of consequences to others as determinants of response inhibition. *J. exper. child Psychol.*, 1965, **2**, 10–30.

|| *CHAPTER EIGHT* ||

DEVELOPMENT AND DYNAMICS: SPECIFIC NEUROTIC REACTIONS

ANXIETY AND PHOBIC REACTIONS

Specific Traumatic Experiences

It is well known that emotionally stressful or traumatic experiences can precipitate all the varieties of neurotic disorder. The most intensively studied cases of this kind are those resulting from war experiences, called shell shock in World War I and combat neuroses or battle fatigue in World War II and later. Grinker and Spiegel (1945) provided a valuable clinical study of behavior disorders of all kinds in Air Force personnel in World War II. It is clear from their findings that some individuals were already highly predisposed to neurotic disorder and only minimal stress was needed to precipitate the disorder. On the basis of retrospective reports the authors concluded that many of these individuals had developed neurotic tendencies within certain family contexts but had found jobs or niches in life, prior to induction in the service, that permitted them to avoid circumstances that would produce the overt neurotic reaction. The inevitable stress of combat, or in some cases precombat training, precipitated the neurotic reaction almost immediately. Other individuals developed neurotic reactions only after unusual specific stress or after long periods of living under chronically stressful conditions. And, of course, many individuals were able to live through acute and chronic stress and not develop crippling neurotic symptoms at all. The most common symptoms were phobic or generalized anxiety reactions. Depression, especially as a concomitant of anxiety, was also common. Conversion and dissociative reactions were relatively rare. In most cases the initial anxiety reactions were closely associated with specific experiences, such as narrowly escaping death in a burning, crashing airplane or having a member of his bomber crew killed before his eyes.

Thus, although war stresses were probably a necessary condition for the neurotic reaction to occur, these stresses were not in most cases a sufficient condition. We still have to explain why, given the same stress experience, some individuals react with neurotic symptoms and some do not. It is generally assumed that the explanation lies in different genetic and past environmental experiences.

If current traumatic experiences in the form of war or natural disaster can produce all the varieties of neurotic disorder, to what extent do less public current or past traumatic experiences account for the origin of the "non-traumatic" adult neuroses? In a theory that he abandoned early in his career Freud proposed that all adult neuroses had their cause in an early childhood sexual trauma. This particular theory is no longer taken seriously, but the role of various kinds of specific traumatic experiences in childhood in the development of adult neurosis remains an important question.

Clinical reports suggest that specific traumatic experiences that produce a strong anxiety response mark the beginning of many phobic reactions. Roberts (1964) studied 41 women who were so phobic about leaving their homes as to be essentially housebound. Twenty-three (60%) readily described specific traumatic experiences related to their first anxiety attacks. One woman's first anxiety reaction occurred when she was standing at a bus stop on the way to visit a friend who had just attempted suicide and whose husband had been making advances to the patient. Three women experienced their first attacks while on the way to visit a child in a hospital for an operation; another, while walking along a street a day or so after her husband's heart attack; another, on receiving a letter telling of her husband's infidelity; etc. Nineteen (50%), however, had had at least one clear-cut neurotic trait, commonly a phobia, in childhood. This suggests that the adult traumatic experience may not have been a sufficient cause in all cases to produce the adult phobia, and that the prior childhood phobia made the women more susceptible to adult phobic reactions. It was not feasible in this study to obtain information about the antecedents of the childhood phobias.

Studies of children and adolescents provide a better source of data than adults on the role of earlier traumatic experiences because they are closer in time to those experiences, and family members, teachers and others can also provide information. Langford (1937), for example, studied 20 children, 16 girls and 4 boys, ages 8–14 years, suffering from acute anxiety attacks. For 16 of the children there were rather definite traumatic experiences preceding the anxiety attacks. In 6 of these children the attacks followed within a month or two after tonsillectomies given under ether anesthetic; in another 6 children there had been either a death in the family or, in 2 cases, the witnessing of rather violent deaths in the neighborhood. In addition to the high incidence of prior traumatic experiences Langford also reported that "they were, with one exception, all timid children who did not mix well with their playmates." The latter finding is consistent with the possibility that genetic influences contributed to the fearfulness which when augmented by the specific traumatic experience yielded the acute anxiety attacks. It is also possible that prior social learning experiences had produced the trait of fearfulness or timidity.

Overprotectiveness and the Development of Fearfulness

The negative affect of fear would seem to be present in many children who come to the attention of mental health clinics and are described as shy, inhibited, anxious, and withdrawn. Parent protectiveness and overcontrol in early childhood may contribute to the development of such characteristics. For example, lack of dominance and assertiveness in children has been found to be related to early mother protectiveness (Kagan & Moss, 1962) and to high parental demands, supervision and consistency (McCord, McCord, & Howeard, 1961).

In studies of clinical populations which mostly used interview-based ratings Jenkins (1968), Lewis (1954), Rosenthal et al. (1959), and Rosenthal et al. (1962) compared parent characteristics of a group of inhibited, anxious neurotic children with a group of aggressive, antisocial children. In all studies, parents of the inhibited children showed greater restrictiveness or protection.

The development of school "phobias" in young children is especially illuminating as an example of the role of parent overprotection in child fearfulness, and as a further example of a neurotic symptom that is best seen as a dyadic system. Eisenberg (1958) and Waldfogel (1957), report findings on clinical studies of such children. These authors conclude, rather convincingly, that in a high proportion of cases the children and their mothers (in a few cases, father) have developed a mutually dependent relationship, where separation is very disturbing to both. Starting to school simply represents the first time that sustained separation is demanded, although there are usually isolated incidents of previous intense anxiety or disturbance on the part of the child when mother has been away temporarily. School phobia is a misnomer in this case. The "phobic situation" might be better described as involving separation from mother.

Eisenberg (1958) studied 11 preschool children (6 boys and 5 girls) with such separation problems in a special nursery school for emotionally disturbed children. Direct observations were made of the mother and child behavior during the early phases of nursery school attendance. During the first days the child remained close to mother and then began to oscillate toward and away from the attractions of the play area. As the child began to look less at mother and move away from her, she would take a seat closer to the child and occasionally use a pretext of wiping his nose or checking his toilet needs for intruding into the child's activity; separation was as difficult for mother as for the child. Similar resistance to separation was shown by the mother when she was required to move to an adjacent room as part of the program for reducing the mutual separation anxiety.

Interviews with the mothers indicated that in most cases the child as an infant had been treated with apprehensive oversolicitude. They were not trusted to babysitters outside the immediate family and later were constantly warned of hazards if they ventured away from home. The circumstances in the mother's life that led to this behavior with her child were varied. For some mothers the child was a late arrival after many sterile years. Some saw the child in terms of their own unhappy childhood and wished to protect the child from similar experiences. Others were frustrated in their marriage relationship and turned to their children for a "secure" relationship. Many mothers were also seen as experiencing angry feelings toward the child, displaced, perhaps, from an unhappy marriage or paradoxically from being tied down so much by the child. The occasional awareness of this anger, or its impulsive expression toward the child, would lead to compensatory protectiveness and greater tightening of the symbiotic bond.

In order to have more confidence in such an analysis of the development of nursery school separation phobias, we would need information about the relevant reinforcement contingencies as they occurred in the past. How did the fear response become associated with separation? It is possible that some fear-arousing incident occurred in association with the mother's leaving that would account for the initial fear-separation association. It seems more likely in the case of Eisenberg's children that the early development of the mother-child symbiotic relationship preceded the fear development. Thus, we might speculate that shortly after birth the mother began the overprotective regime that fostered an unusually close attachment and dependency upon her. This overprotective behavior on the mother's part might have any of the several sources noted above. For purposes of this analysis it does not matter what motivates the mother. We only assume that the independent or separative tendencies on the part of the child are aversive to the mother and consequently any reduction of such tendencies is reinforcing to her. Under such a regime the child is increasingly likely to turn to mother for help and as a source of "positive affect" to reduce all sources of "negative affect" such as bodily hurts, illnesses, and teasing by other children. The child eventually learns to coerce mother into providing "mothering" at the onset of any disturbing situation by emitting the first signs of distress—a whimper, a few tears, a yell, etc. One result of such a system is that the child does not learn to successfully master new fear experiences. Both humans and animals can be observed to master mild to moderate fear in new situations by repeatedly approaching and withdrawing from the feared situation. The repeated arousal of the fear response in small, controlled doses in this way leads eventually to extinction of the fear response. The overprotected child is not allowed to learn the skills involved in mastering new fears in this way and is in danger of being overwhelmed at some future time by an unavoidable fear arousing situation. The high prevalence of transitory fears in normal children (Jersild & Holmes, 1935) suggests that no special circumstances have to be hypothesized to account for some degree of initial fearfulness. The important factor is whether or not the child is able to master the fears that would seem to be inevitably present.

An abrupt separation of the mother from an overprotected child might well lead to an emotional reaction in the child with a strong fear component. No additional fear-evoking circumstances would have to be present. Once a fear reaction of high intensity had occurred, it could by classical conditioning become more strongly associated with circumstances of separation. If the fear were also reduced by the mother's return, then clinging to the mother as a response to fear would also be reinforced. Overt manifestations of fear on the child's part would likely become discriminative stimuli for the mother's protective behavior. In addition to the factors involved in the above formulation, the mother may also further strengthen the separation-fear association by verbal means; for example, by frequent warnings about the various dangers that lie in wait away from mother. It is also possible that the fear could be maintained to some extent as an instrumental response with reinforcement in the form of mother's comforting.

Although the above formulation may seem reasonable, it should be emphasized that it is based on very indirect sources of data. Formulations of this kind can be made to appear simple and elegant as long as we do not ask for their confirmation by direct measures. Then frequently the whole business turns out to be more complicated than the theory implies. For example, careful description of the child's response to separation might reveal that, in some cases, the child is not responding with fear at all but with temper-tantrum-like behavior including crying and other signs of distress. The absence of strong fear would suggest some differences in the past reinforcement contingencies leading to the disorder and also some differences in treatment strategies. It is more likely, for example, that tantrum-like behavior would be learned primarily as an instrumental response aimed at coercing certain kinds of parent behavior, rather than as a classically conditioned emotional response.

Instrumental and Observational Learning in the Development of Anxiety

The role of instrumental learning and observational learning in the development of anxiety is not as obvious as the classical conditioning process, and deserves further consideration. Can, in fact, anxiety be learned on the basis of either observational or instrumental learning processes? Thus far the instigation of anxiety by certain aversive experiences and the possible classical conditioning of these emotional reactions to other stimuli has been emphasized. If a child observes a parent or sibling react with fear, will he imitate this response? As mentioned in Chapter 5, there is experimental evidence that shows vicarious conditioning of autonomic responses will occur when young adult subjects observe other subjects supposedly being shocked and reacting with pain (Bandura & Rosenthal, 1966; Berger, 1962). It was emphasized that vicarious conditioning of this kind is based on the prior learning of empathic emotional responses to overt signs of distress shown by other person, or to mediating cognitive representations of the expected effects of a given experience on another person. If an empathic fear response has been learned, this learning would provide an important basis on which the child might learn fear, or other negative affect responses, to new stimuli as a result of simply observing another person's expressive reactions to those stimuli. Or, again assuming prior learning, the child may respond to another person's verbal statements about being afraid in a certain situation with a fear reaction of his own.

The further strengthening of a negative affect response by subsequent reinforcement may also occur. There is experimental evidence that individuals can learn to modify certain autonomic responses such as heart rate (Engel and Hanson, 1966; Lang, Sroufe, and Hastings, 1967; Shearn, 1962) and GSR (Crider, Shapiro and Tursky, 1966) in response to external reinforcement. Some people can learn to use, for example, an increase in heart rate as an instrumental response to achieve a reinforcement in the same way that a person might learn to use motor behavior to achieve reinforcements. The evidence for instrumental learning of autonomic responses, however, indicates that this is not an easy task, and that most individuals have difficulty with this kind of learning. It remains questionable to what extent a strong fear response, with its associated unpleasantness, would often be acquired or maintained on the basis of instrumental learning. Other forms of emotional reaction, such as grief, are more readily controlled and less aversive, and probably serve as instrumental responses to achieve reinforcements more often than fear. A child, for example, might well learn to cry in order to obtain parental attention and comforting, to avoid parental criticisms, or to avoid some unpleasant task.

Avoidance Strategies and Anxiety

Irrationality of anxiety reactions. It has been commonly assumed, especially in the psychoanalytic tradition, that a person who experiences neurotic anxiety reactions is not aware of the "real" sources of the anxiety. There is probably some truth in this although it is unlikely that an unresolved oedipal conflict represents the "real" source of anxiety in many cases. The "real" sources are probably some combination of genetic predispositions, specific traumatic incidents, and social learning experiences as just discussed. The anxiety reaction is nevertheless frequently experienced as irrational and not clearly related to anything. Another way of saying the same thing is that the person cannot specify and is presumably unaware of the discriminative stimuli that elicit the anxiety reaction.

Before invoking learned avoidance strategies as an explanation, it should be pointed out that we are probably incapable of clearly specifying many discriminative stimuli that affect our behavior. An experiment (Latané & Darley, 1968) in social psychology illustrates this point. The subjects, seated in a small room, faced an ambiguous but potentially critical situation as a stream of smoke began to pour into the room through a wall vent. In one condition each subject was alone in the room; in another three subjects were together. Eighteen out of 24 subjects in the Alone condition reported the smoke to some authority, whereas only 1 out of 27 subjects in the Together condition reported the smoke. Despite this dramatic effect of the experimental manipulation of being alone or together, subjects in the Together condition almost invariably reported that they paid little or no attention to the reactions of other people in the room. It is possible that they were aware of the effect of the presence of other people on their behavior, and were unwilling to admit it. It seems more likely, however, that they were simply unaware that the other people represented discriminative stimuli that affected their behavior.

The inability to clearly specify contingencies between stimuli and responses does not have to involve a learned avoidance of being aware of the contingencies. After all it takes a fair amount of effort, and perhaps training, to become competent at identifying these contingencies. Unless one is reinforced for doing this, why bother? Thus some of the irrationality of anxiety reactions may simply involve this general lack of clarity about contingencies.

Nevertheless, it is also likely that individuals do develop not-think-about responses with respect to the central features of the original anxiety arousing circumstances. These responses would serve to avoid some anxiety arousing thoughts, such as memories, but would not prevent external stimuli associated with the original circumstances from either directly eliciting anxiety or stimulating thoughts that would elicit anxiety.

Displacement in phobias. It was not necessary to assume that any displacement had occurred in the school phobias described by Eisenberg (1958) and referred to earlier in this chapter. Separation from mother remained the phobic stimulus throughout the development of the phobia. In the psychoanalytic tradition, however, the phobic reaction is considered to represent a displacement of anxiety from the oedipal conflict to the phobic object. In the case of Little Hans described by Freud in 1909 (1950) Little Hans' fear of being bitten by horses was interpreted as a displacement of the fear of castration by his father.

The displacement of fear, or negative affect, seems to involve a different mechanism than the displacement of behaviors such as aggression. It may be recalled that in Chapter 5 displacement was considered to result when the expression of a behavioral tendency such as aggression toward a specific person was associated with an aversive consequence. The aggressive response might then be displaced along a dimension of stimulus similarity to objects where a less aversive consequence would be associated with its expression. The negative affect in this case is "causing" the displacement but is not itself being displaced. The displacement theory of phobias, however, suggests that the fear itself is being displaced.

It seems more likely that aspects of the phobic object were actually present at the time of the initial anxiety reactions and acquired their anxiety eliciting power on the basis of classical conditioning. In Roberts' (1964) study, for example, most of the agoraphobic women had experienced an anxiety attack in an open street at the onset of their phobic reactions. Rachman and Costello (1961) and Wolpe and Rachman (1960) further substantiate from clinical reports the common occurrence of an anxiety reaction in association with the phobic-object-to-be at the beginning of the disorder. As in the case of anxiety reactions the irrationality of the phobic reaction could result from simple lack of effort and skill in identifying contingencies plus some not-think-about responses to avoid thoughts and memories about the original circumstances.

It is also possible that anxiety might, by stimulus generalization, be aroused by stimuli similar to those present at the original anxiety attack.

Either external stimuli or internal stimuli (thoughts, etc.) might provide dimensions of stimulus generalization. But stimulus generalization gradients always decrease as a function of distance from the target stimulus, and it is at least implied in proposals of fear displacement that the fear to the phobic object is as strong as toward the original source. Empirically it is true that phobic fears can be quite intense.

Whether fear can be displaced to other stimuli in more than a stimulus generalization sense is questionable. Epstein, however, (1962) reports findings consistent with the possibility that fear may come to be stronger at some point on a stimulus generalization dimension than to the target stimulus. Four groups of sport parachutists with varying degrees of jumping experience (1, 5–8, 25–50, and 100 previous jumps) were presented a word-association test just before a jump. The words were grouped in four categories in terms of their relevance to parachuting. Examples in order of increasing relevance are "music," "sky," "fall," and "ripcord." GSR responses to these words increased in magnitude as a function of increasing relevance for the novice group (1 previous jump), but showed an inverted-V-shaped curve for the more experienced parachutists, peaking at the medium or low relevant words. Additional subjects were studied longitudinally; the shifting of the peak response from the most relevant to less relevant words was also demonstrated in each subject. See Figure 11 for an example of such a shift.

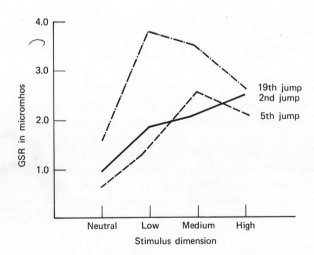

FIGURE 11. **GSR curves at three levels of experience for Subject 1 (Epstein, 1962).**

These results suggest that the fear response is in some way being displaced from the most relevant stimuli. Epstein proposes two factors to account for this finding: 1) the magnitude of the fear response to all related stimuli increases with the repeated fear arousals associated with successive jumps. This factor implies little or no habituation of the fear response to repeated jumps. 2) avoidance responses are learned to reduce the fear associated with the most relevant stimuli. The avoidance responses (denial, intellectualization, substitution of other affects such as anger) outweigh the increases in fear to the most relevant stimuli and a net decrease results at that point. Avoidance responses are not employed, at least as soon or as effectively, for more remote stimuli, and there is a net increase in fear to the more remote stimuli after repeated experiences.

Whether this theory and these findings are directly relevant to phobia formations remains to be seen, but they are suggestive of a possible contributing mechanism. In Epstein's study the repeated fear-arousing experience of parachuting is necessary for the displacement to occur. There is no evidence, however, to suggest that the specific original circumstances of phobic fear induction are repeated on a number of occasions. Strong fear which is slow to extinguish can, however, be learned on the basis of one intense experience, and may provide a basis for future repetitions of the fear response to stimuli that had been present during the original experience. Repetitions would, then, provide the opportunity for the mechanisms proposed by Epstein to produce the displaced phobic response.

OBSESSIVE-COMPULSIVE REACTION

Conflict in Obsessive-Compulsive Disorders

The features of psychological conflict are especially highlighted in the obsessive-compulsive disorder. An intense approach-avoidance conflict is almost invariably present, and is handled by displacements, intellectualization, and other avoidance strategies. It is hypothesized that childhood experiences which would promote such an intense conflict lie behind the development of obsessive-compulsive symptoms, but empirical studies are lacking. Individual studies of clinical cases, however, are consistent with the proposal that as a child the person experienced strong negative affect induction combined with parental reactions designed to produce strong inhibitions.

Persistence of Obsessive Thoughts, A Paradox?

On the surface the repeated experiencing of certain obsessive thoughts, such as killing or injuring someone, would seem to contradict the reinforcement principle. If a thought is unpleasant or aversive why would the person not learn to avoid having this thought as the result of reinforcement associated with removal of an aversive stimulus? Several possibilities might account for the empirical fact that such obsessions do persist.

1. The person has somehow learned to experience the thought without emotional responses so that negative affect is minimized. The discussion in Chapter 6, p. 93, on intellectualization is relevant to this point. This is not a completely satisfactory answer because many patients do report some degree of discomfort associated with their repetitive obsessive thoughts.

2. The obsessive thought may persist in part because it is simply a very strong response that is continually being stimulated by prevailing stimuli. Obsessional thoughts of murder and injury may be continually elicited by the circumstances of a person's marriage or family relationships. Attempts to cope with such a strong response by learned avoidance strategies are only partially successful and thus the recurring response.

3. Sometimes it seems as though the person actively ruminates about the disturbing possibilities, that is, goes out of his way to think about them. In this case there may be an element of do-it-yourself desensitization therapy involved. Wolpe (1958) developed a treatment procedure for phobias called systematic desensitization in which the individual visualizes scenes that become progressively more like the phobic situation. During the visualizations a response incompatible with anxiety, such as deep relaxation, is produced. This method is thought to represent a form of counter-conditioning in which the anxiety is eventually replaced by relaxation. In the case of obsessions it may be that the person permits himself to experience the anxiety arousing thought and occasionally, under circumstances where he is feeling particularly relaxed or having a positive affective experience, the anxiety associated with the thought is partially counter-conditioned or extinguished. This would provide a reinforcement for repeating the obsessive thought on future occasions. Unfortunately the "do-it-yourself" procedure is not set up to carry the program through systematically to successful completion. The anxiety is reinstated from time to time when the thoughts occur under less benign circumstances. Thus the person is on a partial reinforcement schedule that maintains the obsessive thought even though the thought frequently elicits considerable anxiety.

The persistence of obsessive thoughts is less of a problem to explain when some degree of displacement is involved. For example, a person whose strong approach-avoidance conflict about aggression is displaced to preoccupation with a philosophical, scientific, or political issue may express aggression by thinking up arguments to cut his intellectual opponents to shreds or otherwise "demolish" them. Displacement, by definition, means that the aggression is being expressed to targets and by responses where the avoidance response is less strong than the aggressive response.

HYSTERIA

Specific Traumatic Experiences

Traumatic experiences frequently play a role in the causation of hysterical reactions, as was true in the cases of Kate Fox (parental conflict, mother running away from home, etc.), Anna O. (attending to dying father), and the ex-soldier with the dissociative reaction (memory of having killed an officer) described in Chapter 2. A number of conversion and dissociative reactions have their start with a slight physical injury that becomes exaggerated and persists long after the original injury would have healed. We still have to explain, however, why some individuals experience these trauma and develop hysterical reactions and others do not.

Social Learning

It is generally accepted that the incidence of hysterical symptoms in western culture has decreased since the days of Charcot and Freud. A common hypothesis to account for this is a presumed change in society's acceptance and reinforcement of such symptoms. In the 19th century there was less sophistication about possible psychological factors, and it may have been easier for patients as well as their physicians and families to uncritically accept the symptom as indicative of physical illness, and provide many reinforcements in the form of attention, sympathy, and relief from responsibility. Repressive Victorian attitudes toward sexuality, including the pretense that childhood sexuality did not exist, may have also contributed to certain kinds of hysterical reactions in which there was a mutual "conspiracy" between adults and children to deny the sexual meaning of certain symptoms.

Consistent with the hypothesis that psychological sophistication may reduce the incidence of hysteria is the general tendency to find somewhat higher rates in low socioeconomic and educational levels of society. Proctor (1958), for example, found that 13 percent of 191 consecutive children seen at the University of North Carolina Medical School Psychiatric Unit were diagnosed hysterical. This was a much higher incidence rate than seemed to exist in other parts of the country at that time. Proctor indicated that the largely rural areas from which these children came were characterized by low economic and educational levels with a strong element of dour, pleasure-inhibiting fundamentalist religion that emphasized the sinful nature of smoking, drinking, and sex. But at the same time children were likely to experience behavioral inconsistency with these verbal preachments on the part of parents and other adults. For example, they might witness parent sexual intercourse or sleep with the opposite sex parent to an advanced age. The combination of overstimulation with strong verbally induced inhibitions and the lack of psychological sophistication probably contributed to the higher incidence of hysteria.

Schuler and Parenton (1943) reported a study that illustrates the development of a hysterical symptom in an individual and subsequently the development of a group manifestation of the symptom in a high school. Helen, one of the more popular girls in her class, began to show the symptom while attending the homecoming dance. She herself did not dance at that time, nor did her father or older brothers, and she maintained that she was simply not interested in dancing. Nevertheless, as was common among her classmates, she did attend the dance as an observer. During the dance she experienced a transitory twitching and jerking of her right leg. There were several circumstances that might have played a role in the onset of this symptom. A few days before the dance obligatory instruction in dancing had begun in her physical education class. Helen avoided these lessons for the first few class meetings, suggesting the presence of a rather strong inhibition about learning to dance. Three days before the homecoming dance the results of the election of the King, Queen, and Court for the High School Carnival Ball were announced. Although she was a senior and fairly prominent among her classmates, she was not elected to any of these positions—positions in which some competence at dancing might be expected. At about the same time Helen was also becoming aware of the success of a rival for the attentions of a prominent senior boy. The boy was a good dancer and Helen's rival was a vivacious girl who tap-danced so skillfully that she had been asked to perform at the Ball.

The twitching-jerking movements of Helen's leg occurred occasionally during the weeks following the homecoming dance, especially when she was under nervous strain of any sort. Many of her classmates became aware of her symptom at this time, and some apparently thought that it might be contagious. About three weeks after the onset of Helen's symptom, two classmates, Millie and Frances, went to a Mardi Gras dance, and at Frances' home after the dance Millie suddenly developed convulsive jerking movements in the chest and neck. Millie attended class the next day during which she continued to manifest these symptoms. On Thursday morning Helen was observed by many students to be experiencing her attacks during an assembly held before the start of classes. During the second class period Frances began to manifest her spasmodic movements which soon became noticeable to the class. She was taken to the infirmary, but in the meantime her friend Geraldine who sat next to her was getting increasingly nervous. In her own words, "First I trembled a little. Then everybody kept saying, 'Look at Geraldine.' And then I started jumping."

The situation rapidly deteriorated at this point. Soon there were a number of crying, excited girls showing various forms of the jerking movements. Excited parents began to arrive to take their children away from whatever strange epidemic seemed to be occurring. School was finally dismissed, and it was several weeks before all the girls, many of whom were kept home, were fully recovered from their symptoms.

The condition seemingly related to the individual development of the symptom in Helen was a rather strong conflict in which learning to dance played a central role. It is likely that the twitching and jerking leg movements were related in some way to movements involved in dancing. Conflict of this kind probably plays a central role in the development of many conversion reactions. Recall the conflict-inducing culture of certain rural areas in North Carolina reported by Proctor, the conflict of Kate Fox (p. 15) with respect to walking outside during the school recess, and the conflict of the young woman whose visual acuity varied markedly (p. 124).

The conditions that would seem to have facilitated the development of group hysteria were first, and perhaps most important, a clear and visible model (Helen) of the behavior; second, reinforcement for the behavior in the form of attention and concern; third, a general increase in the excitement or arousal level accompanied by expectations that dramatic happenings were in the offing; and fourth, a lack of psychological sophistication. These also would appear to be the conditions, for example, in which faith healings, speaking in tongues, trancelike states, and convulsive seizures are induced in certain religious groups.

Hypnosis and Hysteria

Since the work of Bernheim and Charcot the close relationship between hypnotically induced reactions and hysterical symptoms has been recognized. The relationship is especially emphasized by the fact that in normal subjects conversion and dissociative reactions can be induced under hypnosis which are difficult to distinguish from their naturally occurring hysterical counterparts. Thus a study of hypnosis might shed light on mechanisms involved in the development of hysteria.

Although the phenomenon of hypnosis remains less than completely understood itself, there is a growing body of evidence suggesting the importance of two aspects of the hypnotic procedure. First, the subject must focus his attention on some very restricted field of experience, especially emphasizing the hypnotist's voice, and second the subject must be motivated to cooperate with the hypnotist in undertaking whatever roles may be subsequently asked of him.

Experiences of a mildly hypnotic nature may occur in everyday life. If the person can achieve a sufficient narrowing of attention and blocking out of most sources of incoming stimulation without the aid of a hypnotist he is well on the way to a temporary fugue or amnesic state. Most of us can remember occasions during which we became completely engrossed in a task, if only for a few seconds or minutes, and subsequently realized, or were told by others, that we had been completely oblivious to many things going on around us. It is also likely that during the "dissociative" experience we were not aware even of ourselves, that is our personal identity.

Conversion symptoms in the form of motor and sensory disturbances may also be facilitated in some way by these states of high concentration and strong motivation to escape from some distressing life circumstance. The reduction of pain by producing a cognitive expectation of pain relief in conjunction with the administration of a placebo pill probably has some similarities to the conversion reaction of analgesia. Hilgard (1969), for example, found that pain could be diminished by suggestion under hypnosis. He induced pain experimentally in normal subjects by *ischemia,* that is, by applying a tourniquet that cuts off the blood supply just below the elbow. Pain increases steadily over the next 30 minutes or so to a point where the subject cannot stand it longer and the tourniquet is removed. Six subjects, selected to be highly hypnotizable, were in counterbalanced order subjected on successive days to the ischemic pain experience under either normal waking conditions or under hypnotic suggestions of analgesia. Under hypnotic analgesia the subjects were able to rid themselves of pain for periods of 18–45 minutes, based on both self-ratings of pain and finger blood pressure in the nonischemic hand. During the normal waking state these same subjects reported strongly increasing pain accompanied by increase in blood pressure, and had to terminate the experiment because of unbearable pain much sooner than in the hypnotic state. In the same study Hilgard also reported substantial reduction in self-reported pain associated with immersion of a forearm in cold water under hypnotic analgesia but not for a condition of hypnosis without the analgesic suggestion. Hypnosis by itself, in other words, was not enough to produce the analgesic effect. Hilgard's study, however, leaves unanswered the question of whether the hypnosis inducing procedure is necessary to achieve this degree of pain reduction. Barber (1961) reviewed hypnosis research and concluded that there was no experimental demonstration of any effects achieved under hypnosis that could not be duplicated by subjects simply given strong suggestions to behave in these various ways in the waking state. It is unfortunate that Hilgard did not include a group given strong suggestions under normal waking conditions that they could and would tolerate the pain.

If it should turn out that pain reduction, and other effects analogous to conversion symptoms, can be produced by strong suggestion in the waking state this does not negate the significance of the findings. It would simply blur the distinction between the hypnotic trance and normal waking state suggestion. A tentative conclusion that might be drawn at this time is that *some* individuals can, by techniques that emphasize the narrowing of attention and blocking out of extraneous sources of stimulation, be made to experience changes in sensory function and altered states of consciousness that are similar, if not indistinguishable, from hysterical symptoms. It is a plausible hypothesis that the same mechanisms are involved in naturally occurring hysterical symptoms, except in this case the person has somehow learned to produce the effect without the help of another person such as a hypnotist.

Neurophysiology and Hysterical Analgesia

Hernandez-Peon et al. (1963) reported a study that suggests possible neurophysiological mechanisms in the development of hysterical analgesia. Six months before the study a 15-year-old girl developed a partial paralysis in her left hand. Seven days later she developed analgesia of the entire left arm from fingers to shoulders and loss of the sense of hot and cold in the lower arm. A single pin prick elicited no pain but repetitive pin pricking evoked a report of normal pin prick pain. There were no other physical or neurological abnormalities.

By attaching electrodes to the scalp it is possible to detect sensory potentials evoked by some incoming sensory signal. Since the evoked sensory potentials in the cortex are weak relative to the other electrical activity and random noise being generated, it is necessary to average recordings obtained on a number of trials. When this is done a reliable indication of the evoked potential can be obtained. In this case a series of 40 individual "pin pricks" was applied by electrical stimulation to first one arm and then the other. The right, nonanalgesic arm produced normal evoked potentials. The left, analgesic arm showed no evoked potential. It is known from animal research that neural pathways descending from the cortex can exert an inhibitory influence on specific incoming sensory pathways. Hernandez-Peon suggests that this inhibitory mechanism may be involved in many conversion reactions. That is, individuals may in some way learn to apply this inhibitory mechanism to incoming pain stimuli.

In this same study it was found that under light barbiturate-induced sleep an evoked potential was obtained from the left arm, and an even larger than normal response was obtained from the right arm. This would seem to contradict the hypothesis that the analgesia was being produced by some kind of learned inhibition, if one assumes that barbiturates exert a generally inhibitory function on the brain. In fact, animal research suggests that, among other things, barbiturate drugs selectively decrease the activation of these inhibitory pathways with the net effect of removing the inhibition. The greater-than-normal response of the right arm is consistent with such a disinhibition effect.

Hernandez-Peon does not mention treatment of this case. The evoked potential procedure would provide a valuable objective measure to use in conjunction with systematic attempts to modify various kinds of conversion or dissociative reactions, or in connection with experimental studies designed to study psychological variables that influence these reactions.

DEPRESSION

Specific Traumatic Experiences

Many neurotic depressive reactions would seem to be precipitated by traumatic experiences involving an interpersonal separation or failure experience. Retrospective research suggests that adult depression is more frequently associated with the loss of a parent during childhood than are other symptoms of psychopathology (Beck, 1967; Brown, 1966; Denneby, 1966; Gay & Tonge, 1967; Hill & Price, 1967; Munroe, 1966). Pitts et al. (1965) and Gregory (1966), on the other hand, did not find such a relationship. Beck (1967) performed one of the best designed studies of this type. He selected a sample of 297 psychiatric patients and categorized them according to severity of depressive reaction by means of a Depression Inventory (shown to have some validity in other research). He found that 27 percent of the high-depressed patients as opposed to 12 percent of the low-depressed patients reported the loss of a parent before the age of 16. This difference held up at different age levels, in male and female patients, and in Negro and white patients. An important feature in this study is that the categorization was not based on traditional psychiatric categories but on the prominence of depression alone. In fact, when diagnostic categories such as neurotic depression, psychotic depression, schizophrenia, etc., were used there was no difference in percentages of parent deaths in childhood.

Social Learning

Anger and depression. Individuals do not always react to death or failure with a neurotic depression. What kind of prior social learning experiences would predispose a person to such a reaction? It is a common clinical observation that a person who reacts to a death with depression has had a conflicted relationship with the deceased. The conflict frequently takes the form of the person having been dependent on another person, but also of having felt intense anger that was not expressed and probably not recognized as such. Fleeting wishes that the person would die or thoughts of inflicting injury on the person might be occasionally experienced.

Nemiah (1961) describes a 34-year-old woman, Barbara T., who was admitted to a hospital with attacks of anxiety and symptoms of depression. Her mother had died two years ago, but she had felt no grief and had been unable to cry at the time. She had always been close to her mother, had needed her continual support, and relied on her for advice and guidance. She found it difficult to emancipate herself from her mother and lived with her until after her thirtieth birthday. She had given up a relationship with one man who had wanted to marry her because she was reluctant to break her ties with her mother. The mother had occasional attacks of grand mal epilepsy, and throughout her life Barbara felt responsible for this illness, and was certain that if she argued or otherwise expressed anger at her mother, she would precipitate a seizure and possibly death. Beneath her surface obedience, helpfulness, and concern about her mother's health were intense feelings of resentment and anger. When her mother did die, the presence of the strong anger seems to have inhibited the normal course of the grief reaction. In the course of psychotherapeutic treatment it is common, although not described in this case, for an individual to go through a normal grieving period *after* he has been able to recognize and express his feelings of anger and resentment at the dead person.

Parkes (1965) interviewed psychiatric patients whose symptoms had come on during the terminal illness of or within six months after the death of a parent, spouse, sibling, or child. He compared their reactions to this loss with the reactions of normal widows as reported by Marris (1958), and described on p. 41 of this book. Although there was some similarity in reaction, the psychiatric patients showed more difficulty in accepting the loss, a greater tendency to blame themselves for the loss, or a greater tendency to blame others for the loss. These findings further support the idea that other reactions of one kind or another are complicating the natural expression and course of the grief reaction.

How can unexpressed anger or any other emotional reaction inhibit the normal course of the grief reaction? In answering this question let us consider again the nature of normal grief. Recall that in Chapter 3 grief was described as an extremely unpleasant emotion and that, initially, individuals tend to protest or otherwise deny the grief-precipitating loss. What happens subsequently in the course of normal grief may be likened to the coping process which children and others use in mastering fear, and which was described earlier in this chapter, p. 131. The bereaved person permits himself to think about the loved person and recall memories of enjoyable occasions in small doses. Each time he will experience the pain of grief, but in time with many approaches and retreats from the grief-inducing associations the emotion of grief will diminish (extinguish) in strength. Freed from this handicapping emotion the person can begin to develop other interests in life. Freud (1957) referred to this process as the work of mourning, an apt phrase for what is indeed an active, self-administered treatment procedure.

Nemiah (1961) describes the process as follows:

> The fabric of memories and associations and feelings that permeate the image of the deceased in the mind of the bereaved survivor does not automatically disappear when the loved person dies. In the process of grieving each of the memories and associations must be revived in the mind's eye; as each is thought of, a fresh wave of grief occurs, which gradually fades. As each separate strand of the fabric of associations is thus worked over, it loses its power to evoke the pain of loss, and the loving attachment to the dead one gradually diminishes until the process is complete and the ghost is laid (p. 153–154).

Two factors that might disrupt such a process are unusually intense grief or grief complicated by the presence of anger and self-blame. In either case the person may avoid grief inducing memories because they stir up unbearable negative affect. In the case of grief complicated by anger, the memories tend to awaken the anger which in turn arouses guilt and self-blame. The individual may employ not-think-about-it responses, develop beliefs that deny the reality of the loss, or use other strategies that avoid the unpleasant affect. The process of grieving is stopped cold, and the person remains in the apathetic, emotionless, unresponsive state that we call depression.

Other factors producing deficits in social reinforcement. Some authors (for example, Ferster, 1965; Patterson & Rosenberry, 1969) have stressed the importance of any kind of severe deficit in sources of social reinforcement as contributing to a depressive reaction. Thus not only death but other circumstances such as poverty, social rejection, an intact family that provides very little in the way of attention and responsiveness, and simply lack of skill in obtaining social reinforcements can produce depression according to these authors. This latter factor may not have been emphasized as much as it should have been in previous analyses of depression. Some individuals simply have not learned how to reinforce others for providing them with social reinforcement. For example, in ordinary conversation most people reinforce the other person by looking at the person, head nodding or smiling, and a verbal response whose style and content indicate interest and enjoyment in the interaction. These are effective reinforcers and can maintain social interaction for some time and increase the probability that the two people will get together on future occasions. A person who for whatever reason does not reinforce others for social interchange is putting them on an extinction schedule, and they will eventually cease to interact with him. As a result his own sources of social reinforcement will dwindle. Or even worse, the individual may respond to other people in ways that are aversive and thus drive them away. He may, for example, dwell endlessly on his own gloomy preoccupations, complain bitterly about life in general, or be irritable and critical toward the person to whom he is talking. A person with low skill in obtaining social reinforcement is thus likely to be on a very lean schedule of social reinforcement. Any new decrease in the availability of social reinforcement, although in absolute magnitude no different from what most other people cope with successfully, represents for him a *relative* decrease of enormous magnitude. And it reduces him to an absolute level of social reinforcement that is indeed low. The more acute symptoms of neurotic depression might occur at this time.

Another circumstance associated with low rates of positive social reinforcement is one in which behavior is largely motivated by avoidance of unpleasant or punishing consequences. Parents, wife, children, friends, teachers, or employers will not like him, may criticize him, divorce him, give him low grades, or fire him if he does not behave in certain ways. When one's life comes to be dominated by aversive control, there is likely to be a major deficit of positive social reinforcement. One no longer does things because they are fun, interesting, and socially rewarding, but because one will be punished if one does not. Such a regimen may well evoke anger and resentment and eventually depression.

Previous depressive reactions. Another factor should probably be added to the above in considering the development of depression; namely, that prior depressive reactions increase the probability that such a reaction will be elicited by similar circumstances in the future. It is proposed that some components of the grief reaction, as is true of fear, can be classically conditioned to stimuli closely associated with the occurrence of the reaction. Thus, if a young child in response to prolonged separation had experienced an intense depressive reaction, in the future similar and less prolonged separations would be more likely to produce a depressive reaction than if the earlier one had not occurred. Repeated occasions of depressive reaction would make it possible for anticipatory thoughts about separation or related events such as loss of money or prestige to become conditioned stimuli for depression. The incipient phases of grief itself could become stimuli that elicit stronger grief.

Self-esteem and depression. We can approach a definition of self-esteem by proposing a dimension at one end of which are individuals who characteristically evaluate their performance negatively, regardless of the objective degree of success, and at the other end are individuals who evaluate their performance positively regardless of the objective degree of success. More is involved, however, than evaluation of performance. A person also develops a cognitive representation of "self," a summary picture of all those characteristics that form "him." Evaluative reactions are learned toward this concept of self so that one can be said to have positive or negative self attitudes, or high or low self-esteem. For most people self-evaluative reactions are not global with respect to either performance or the self-concept. That is, a person positively values certain aspects of himself and negatively values other aspects.

Some individuals, especially depressed people, do have rather global negative self-evaluations that are applied to their total self-concept; they believe they are no good, unworthy, and incompetent. If such a person does succeed at something, he is likely to interpret his success as just luck, believe that he will surely fail next time, or maintain that the task did not measure anything important. This cognition or belief may be very resistant to change. The interpretation of ambiguous situations as failures or rejections, or the interpretation of small failures and criticisms as major failures and devastating criticisms can probably maintain a depressive reaction.

What are some of the factors that might contribute to the development of low self-esteem? Since the low self-esteem person reacts with expectations of failure and subsequent self-criticisms that are not contingent on external standards of performance, it is a likely hypothesis that he has experienced much disapproval from others in the past that was not contingent on some reasonable criterion of successful performance. One contributing factor would be parents who have responded indiscriminately with disapproval in a manner independent of the child's actual successes and failures. This may take many forms. For example, a child may bring home a report card that shows some improvement in reading. The parent may start off by giving some praise for this improvement but immediately launch into a lecture about bringing the other grades up, why had he not been doing better all along, etc., so that the subsequent lecture turns the overall parent response into an aversive statement of disapproval. In some cases the parents may have set unreasonably high standards so that for all practical purposes the child experiences nothing but disapproval over the range of variation of his relative successes and failures. After noncontingent disapproval has been experienced for a number of years, one would expect future occasions in which performance is evaluated to elicit expectations of failure and disapproval. Of course reality factors such as intelligence level, physical defect, or body build may affect the proportion of positive evaluations received and thus affect self-esteem. In assessing the role of parent-child interaction in the development of self-esteem we will assume that these reality factors are constant.

Verbalizations of self-criticism may be reinforced by the parents. This is similar to the reinforcement of the confession response. In this case the child is reinforced for saying that he is incompetent or otherwise blameworthy. The reinforcement may take the form of the parent ceasing to make aversive critical comments after the child makes the desired statement. Thus, the child learns to "beat the parent to the punch" by criticizing himself before the parent has a chance to criticize him. Such self-administered criticisms also may be preferable because they give the child some control over the giving of punishment as opposed to the uncertainty of future parent punishment of an unknown intensity. Pervin (1963), for example, has found that subjects prefer self-administered as opposed to experimenter-administered shocks.

Overt and covert verbalizations of self-criticism may also be learned on the basis of their association with punishment termination. Aronfreed (1964) found that children verbalized a specific self-critical reaction to transgression when the experimenter had used this specific critical response on previous occasions at the termination of punishment rather than at the beginning of punishment. Aronfreed proposed that past associations between transgression and subsequent punishment make it likely that future transgressions will elicit anxiety about the expected punishment. The parent, or other punisher, has in the past made critical comments about the child's misbehavior while administering the punishment, and these critical comments by virtue of their association with the *cessation of punishment* acquire secondary reinforcing properties. In the future the child learns to make these self-critical comments soon after a transgression because they serve to reduce the anxiety about anticipated punishment.

It should be emphasized that there is no necessary relationship between the learning of self-critical responses in this way and self-regulatory behavior aimed at improving performance or resisting temptation. It is quite possible for learning contingencies to be such that the child repeatedly transgresses or otherwise falls short of some standard of performance *and* continually makes self-critical statements. In the discussion of self-regulation it was suggested that thoughts of parental disapproval (criticism) with associated negative affect could serve as a source of self-reinforcement for avoiding transgressions. How do thoughts of criticism in one case lead to behavioral control and not in the other? The answer may be that it is necessary for the learning contingencies to be such that the child learns to make the self-critical thought *before* the transgression occurs rather than afterwards.

One final factor that could contribute to the development of low self-esteem would be a parent with low self-esteem who provides a model for the child to imitate.

Empirical research on child rearing antecedents of self-esteem has been meager. Coopersmith (1967) reports a study directly related to child rearing antecedents of self-esteem in 10- to 12-year old boys that involved a variety of measures of child self-esteem. The validity of these measures was supported by several experiments using behavioral measures. Parent variables were largely limited to mother self-reports derived from an interview and a questionnaire. High self-esteem children were found to have higher IQ's, to be more well formed and coordinated physically, to come less often from broken homes, and to have a strong but nonsignificant tendency to come from higher socioeconomic backgrounds. These "reality" characteristics could easily increase expectations of success and probably influenced the author's measure of self-esteem. It is unfortunate that high and low self-esteem groups were not matched on these variables in order to study the unconfounded effects of child rearing variables.

The child rearing results are nevertheless of some interest in that they parallel the results obtained by Baumrind (1967) on 3- to 4-year-old children described earlier. On the basis of mother interview ratings Coopersmith found mothers of high self-esteem boys to have higher self-esteem themselves, to be more satisfied with the father's child rearing practices, to have less conflict with the father, to have higher rapport (a friendly, mutually satisfying relationship) with her son, to demand higher standards of performance, to enforce rules and demands with consistency and firmness, to use reasoning and discussion rather than arbitrary, punitive discipline, and to use more rewards and less punishment in training the child. Baumrind found most of these characteristics to be associated with parents of her energetic–friendly group and the opposite to be true for parents of the conflicted–irritable group.

These results are more or less consistent with the factors proposed as contributing to low self-esteem. However, Coopersmith's low self-esteem boys probably represent a generally maladjusted and somewhat disadvantaged (in terms of IQ, physical build and family stability) group in which low self-esteem is only one of several traits reflecting psychological disturbance. If this is the case the parent traits are not necessarily related to son self-esteem in a highly specific way.

Multiple determinants of depression. There is no one kind of social learning experience associated with the development of depression. Depression may result from various combinations of the factors discussed above, a conflicted relationship with a deceased person, severe deficits in available social reinforcements, lack of skill in social interaction, aversive control of behavior, previous depressive reactions, and conditions producing low self-esteem. As is true for most neurotic disorders we need more research on the way these proposed factors may actually contribute to the development of depression.

TREATMENT OF NEUROTIC DISORDER

It is not possible to provide an intensive critique of treatment procedures within the limits of this book. The psychoanalytic technique developed by Freud, various modifications of this technique developed by the neo-Freudians, and other approaches, such as the client-centered therapy of Carl Rogers, have been widely used in the treatment of neurotic disorders. Methodologically sound research is rare, but a reasonable conclusion at this time is that *some* (presumably the more skilled) therapists help *some* neurotic patients. Considering all therapists and all individuals who have been treated it is likely that the overall effects have been relatively weak, albeit expensive and time consuming.

Several trends in recent years are cause for some optimism in the treatment of neurotic disorders. There is, for example, an increasing tendency to involve the whole family directly in the treatment process when one or more members has neurotic symptoms. If family interaction does indeed play an important role in the development of neurotic disorders, these family-oriented approaches make a great deal of sense. Another new vogue in recent years has been the advent of the behavioral therapies. For one such procedure, systematic desensitization, there is increasing research support for the conclusion that it is more effective (and efficient in terms of time) than the older psychotherapies in treating restricted phobias (Land et al., 1965; Paul, 1966). The virtue of the behavioral therapies is not necessarily in their proven worth, however, but rather that they lend themselves to systematic research which can sift and winnow the effective ingredients of therapy from the nonessentials.

CONCLUDING COMMENTS

This brings us to the end of our consideration of neurotic disorders, and certain broad conclusions might be reemphasized. Neurosis is not a single entity, but refers rather to a spectrum of psychological handicaps caused by a variety of biological and social factors. The relative weighing of biological factors, the social learning history (especially in the family) and immediate situational experiences will vary from person to person. In most cases the biological (hereditary or otherwise) and social learning factors interact in such a way as to make impossible a decision about which is the primary cause. And many neurotic symptoms can best be seen as part of an interacting system between two or more people.

Much remains to be learned about neurotic disorders, especially in terms of the family interaction patterns associated with their early development. There are only a handful of studies in this area that go beyond the individual case study type of approach and employ behaviorally oriented measures of family interaction. Future studies of this kind should greatly aid in the development of treatment procedures. In time, perhaps, we can devise preventive measures to reduce the incidence of these destructive and handicapping disorders, and thus "free" a greater proportion of future generations to more fully develop their human potentials.

REFERENCES

Aronfreed, J. The origin of self-criticism. *Psychol. Rev.*, 1964, **71**, 193–218.

Bandura, A., & Rosenthal, T. L. Vicarious classical conditioning as a function of arousal level. *J. pers. soc. Psychol.*, 1966, **3**, 54–62.

Barber, T. X. Physiological effects of "hypnosis." *Psychol. Bull.*, 1961, **58**, 390–419.

Baumrind, D. Child care practices anteceding three patterns of preschool behavior. *Genetic Psychol. Monogr.*, 1967, **75**, 43–88.

Beck, A. T. *Depression.* New York: Harper and Row, 1967.

Berger, S. M. Conditioning through vicarious instigation. *Psychol. Rev.*, 1962, **69**, 450–466.

Brown, F. Childhood bereavement and subsequent psychiatric disorder. *Brit. J. Psychiat.*, 1966, **112**, 1035–1041.

Coopersmith, S. *The antecedents of self-esteem.* San Francisco: W. H. Freeman, 1967.

Crider, A., Shapiro, D., & Tursky, B. Reinforcement of spontaneous electrodermal activity. *J. comp. physiol. Psychol.*, 1966, **61**, 20–27.

Denneby, C. M. Childhood bereavement and psychiatric illness. *Brit. J. Psychiat.*, 1966, **112**, 1049–1069.

Eisenberg, L. School phobia: A study in the communication of anxiety. *Amer. J. Psychiat.*, 1958, **114**, 712–718.

Engel, B. T., & Hanson, S. P. Operant conditioning of heart rate slowing. *Psychophysiology*, 1966, **3**, 176–187.

Epstein, S. The measurement of drive and conflict in humans: Theory and experiment. In M. R. Jones (Ed.), *Nebraska symposium on motivation.* Lincoln, Neb.: University of Nebraska Press, 1962.

Ferster, C. B. Classification of behavioral pathology. In L. Krasner and L. P. Ullman (Eds.), *Research in behavior modification.* New York: Holt, Rinehart and Winston, 1965.

Freud, S. *Collected papers,* Vol. III. London: Hogarth Press, 1950.

Gay, M. J., & Tonge, W. L. The late effects of loss of parents in childhood. *Brit. J. Psychiat.,* 1967, **113,** 753–759.

Gregory, I. W. Retrospective data concerning childhood loss of a parent. II: Category of parental loss by decade of birth, diagnosis and MMPI. *Arch. Gen. Psychiat.,* 1966, **15,** 362–367.

Grinker, R. R., & Spiegel, J. P. *Men under stress.* New York: McGraw-Hill Book Co., 1945.

Hernandez-Peon, R., Chavez-Ibarra, G., & Aguilar-Figueroa, E. Somatic evoked potentials in one case of hysterical anesthesia. *E.E.G. & clin. Neurophysiol.,* 1963, **15,** 889–892.

Hilgard, E. R. Pain as a puzzle for psychology and physiology. *Amer. Psychologist,* 1969, **24,** 103–113.

Hill, O. W., & Price, J. S. Childhood bereavement and adult depression. *Brit. J. Psychiat.,* 1967, **113,** 743–751.

Jenkins, R. L. The varieties of children's behavioral problems and family dynamics. *Amer. J. Psychiat.,* 1968, **124,** 1440–1445.

Jersild, A. T., & Holmes, F. B. Children's fears. *Child Develop. Monogr.,* 1935, No. 20.

Kagan, J., & Moss, H. A. *Birth to maturity: A study in psychological development.* New York: Wiley, 1962.

Lang, P. J., Lazovik, A. D., & Reynolds, D. J. Desensitization, suggestibility and pseudotherapy. *J. abnorm. soc. Psychol.,* 1965, **70,** 395–402.

Lang, P. J., Sroufe, L. A., & Hastings, J. E. Effects of feedback and instructional set on the control of cardiac-rate variability. *J. exp. Psychol.,* 1967, **75,** 425–431.

Langford, W. Anxiety attacks in children. *Amer. J. Orthopsychiat.,* 1937, **7,** 210–219.

Latané, B., & Darley, J. M. Group inhibition of bystander intervention in emergencies. *J. pers. soc. Psychol.,* 1968, **10,** 215–221.

Lewis, H. *Deprived children.* London: Oxford University Press, 1954.

McCord, W., McCord, J., & Howard, A. Familial correlates of aggression in nondelinquent male children. *J. abnorm. soc. Psychol.,* 1961, **62,** 79–83.

Munro, A. Parental deprivation in depressive patients. *Brit. J. Psychiat.,* 1966, **112,** 443–457.

Nemiah, J. C. *Foundations of Psychopathology.* New York: Oxford University Press, 1961.

Parkes, C. M. Bereavement and mental illness. Part 1. A clinical study of the grief of bereaved psychiatric patients; and Part 2. A classification of bereavement reactions. *Brit. J. Med. Psychiat.,* 1965, **38,** 1–12, 13–26.

Patterson, G. R., & Rosenberry, C. A social learning formulation of depression. Paper presented at International Conference on Behavior Modification, Banff, Alberta, 1969.

Paul, G. L. *Insight vs. desensitization in psychotherapy.* Stanford, Calif.: Stanford University Press, 1966.

Pervin, L. A. The need to predict and control under conditions of threat. *J. Pers.,* 1963, **31,** 570–587.

Pitts, F. N., Jr., Meyer, J., Brooks, M., & Winokur, G. Adult psychiatric illness assessed for childhood parental loss, and psychiatric illness in family members—a study of 748 patients and 250 controls. *Amer. J. Psychiat.*, 1965, Suppl. 121: i–x.

Proctor, J. T. Hysteria in childhood. *Amer. J. Orthopsychiat.*, 1958, **28**, 394–406.

Rachman, S., & Costello, C. G. The aetiology and treatment of children's phobias: A review. *Amer. J. Psychiat.*, 1961, **118**, 97–105.

Roberts, A. H. Housebound housewives—A follow-up study of a phobic anxiety state. *Brit. J. Psychiat.*, 1964, **110**, 191–197.

Rosenthal, M. J., Finkelstein, M., Ni, E., & Berkwitz, G. K. A study of mother-child relationships in the emotional disorders of children. *Genetic Psychol. Monogr.*, 1959, **60**, 65–116.

Rosenthal, M. J., Ni, E., Finkelstein, M., & Berkwitz, G. H. Father-child relationships and children's problems. *AMA Arch. gen. Psychiat.*, 1962, **7**, 360–373.

Schuler, E. A., & Parenton, V. J. A recent epidemic of hysteria in a Louisiana High School. *J. soc. Psychol.*, 1943, **17**, 221–235.

Shearn, D. W. Operant conditioning of heart rate. *Science*, 1962, **137**, 530–531.

Waldfogel, S. The development, meaning, and management of school phobia. *Amer. J. Orthopsychiat.*, 1957, **27**, 754–780.

Wolpe, J. *Psychotherapy by reciprocal inhibition.* Stanford, Calif.: Stanford University Press, 1958.

Wolpe, J., & Rachman, S. Psychoanalytic evidence: A critique based on Freud's case of Little Hans. *J. nerv. ment. Dis.*, 1960, **131**, 135–148.

AUTHOR INDEX

SUBJECT INDEX